Current Topics in Infection
General Editor: Professor Ian Phillips

Titles now published

Forthcoming titles

Genital infection by *Chlamydia trachomatis*

J. D. Oriel, MD

Director, Department of Genito-urinary medicine,
University College Hospital, London

G. L. Ridgway, MD, BSc, MRCPath

Consultant Medical Microbiologist, University College Hospital,
London

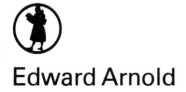

Edward Arnold

©J. D. Oriel and G. L. Ridgway 1982

First published 1982
by Edward Arnold (Publishers) Ltd
41 Bedford Square, London WC1B 3DQ

British Library Cataloguing in Publication Data
Oriel, J. D.
  Genital infection by Chlamydia trachomatis.
  (Current topics in infection, ISSN 0260-1664; 2)
  1. Communicable diseases
  2. Genito-urinary organs – Diseases
  I. Title II. Ridgway, G. L. III. Series
  616.6   RC871
  ISBN 0-7131-4376-2

Set in 10/11pt Linoterm Baskerville by The Castlefield Press of Northampton
and printed in Great Britain by Butler and Tanner Ltd, Frome and London

Preface

Sexually transmitted diseases are common, and there have been many attempts to control them. In general, the greatest efforts have been against the classical 'venereal diseases' syphilis and gonorrhoea, but in many societies (including our own) these infections are outnumbered by an important group of diseases, non-gonococcal urethritis and its related syndromes.

A major cause of these disorders is *Chlamydia trachomatis*. This parasite has been known for over seventy years. Some strains are responsible for the familiar blinding disease trachoma, but others (with which we are concerned in this book) are associated with a wide range of genital tract and related ocular diseases.

It is not always realised that *C. trachomatis* is an important genital pathogen and has the potential to cause as much disease in men, women and infants as *Neisseria gonorrhoeae*. In this volume we have attempted to describe the organism and some of its major effects. If we have discussed the microbiology at length, it is because we think it is fundamental to the understanding of pathogenesis, and because we have found that close collaboration between clinic and laboratory is essential for the diagnosis and effective treatment of chlamydial infections.

We have described the genital and other diseases associated with these organisms in what we hope is adequate detail, but the literature on the subject is enormous and we do not claim that this is a comprehensive review. Neither of us is an ophthalmologist, and our colleague Mr J. H. Kelsey, Consultant Ophthalmologist to University College Hospital, has kindly read the sections on chlamydial eye disease.

In a rapidly developing subject opinions change or may be discarded, and some topics are controversial. We have tried to deal dispassionately with these, but we have not shrunk from expressing our own views. Indeed, many of these have been modified as we have written the book.

We are grateful to our clinical and laboratory staff for their co-operation over many years, to Mr P. Luton for the photographs, and to our publishers for their patience.

London 1981   JDO
                                                     GLR

Contents

1

Introduction

The Ebers papyrus (1500 BC) contains a description of an exudative cicatrizing eye disease, and the application of copper salts is recommended for therapy. This disease was already known to the Chinese, and in ancient Greece and Rome there were many notable sufferers, including Paul of Tarsus, Cicero, Horace and Pliny the Younger. The term **trachoma**, which means rough eye, was coined by Pedanius Diascarides, a Sicilian physician, in 60 AD. By the following year Galen had delineated the four stages of the disease. Trachoma spread from the Middle East across Europe, carried by the Crusaders returning from the Holy Land, and the Egyptian campaigns of Napoléon Bonaparte led to a second wave of infection in Europe.

The genital syndromes associated with *C. trachomatis* may also have an ancient history. In Leviticus (Chapter 15, vv. 1–2) we read 'And the Lord spake unto Moses and to Aaron, saying "Speak unto the children of Israel and say unto them, when any man hath a running issue of his flesh, because of this issue he is unclean"'. This is followed by somewhat draconian advice on epidemiological control. This passage is often cited as an early reference to gonorrhoea, but could equally apply to non-gonococcal urethritis (NGU).

Neisser discovered the gonococcus in 1879, and Gram's staining method was described soon afterwards. In the 1880s the use of Gram staining and culture systems for the gonococcus showed the existence of gonococcal and non-gonococcal forms of urethritis. Ophthalmia neonatorum was very common at this time, and it soon became plain that there were gonococcal and non-gonococcal forms of this disease as well. Kroner (1884) suggested that non-gonococcal ophthalmia might be caused by an unknown infective agent in the maternal genital tract.

In 1883 the first study of the aetiology of trachoma appeared when Koch described the recovery of *Haemophilus aegyptius* and *N. gonorrhoeae* from patients with 'Egyptian ophthalmia', a disease synonymous with trachoma, but the real cause was not revealed until the work of Halberstaedter and von Prowazek was published in 1907. They described the intraepithelial inclusions which now bear their name in conjunctival scrapings from experimentally infected orang-utans. Two years later they described similar inclusions in conjunctival smears from babies with non-gonococcal ophthalmia.

Heyman (1910) saw inclusions in cervical and urethral cells from the parents of babies with ophthalmia neonatorum, but some of the cases were also infected with the gonococcus, leading to confusion and controversy. Post-gonococcal urethritis (PGU) was stated by von Wahl (1911) not to be due to gonorrhoea, but to result from a primary mixed infection with gonorrhoea and an agent of NGU.

A firm link between ocular and genital infections by *C. trachomatis* was established by Fritsch, Hofstätter and Lindner (1910), who inoculated the conjunctivae of monkeys with scrapings from the eyes of babies with chlamydial ophthalmia, cervical secretions from their mothers, and urethral secretions from men with NGU. In each case, the monkeys developed inclusion conjunctivitis, with identical pathology, irrespective of the source of the inoculum. Thus within a few years the key facts of the epidemiology of genital chlamydial infection — its association with NGU, its sexual transmission, and the ocular involvement of neonates — had been discovered.

Further major advances were constricted by the failure of researchers to culture *C. trachomatis* in the laboratory. Sporadic reports of the involvement of chlamydiae in both ocular and genital infection appeared, some confirmed by transmission of the disease to the conjunctivae of the eyes of blind human volunteers. Inadvertent human to human transmission was described; for example a gynaecologist splashed in the eye with blood during a dilatation and curettage developed inclusion conjunctivitis (Thygeson and Mengert, 1936); and ocular infection of a nurse acquired whilst treating a baby with inclusion conjunctivitis was described.

Similarities between the life cycle of *C. psittaci* and *C. trachomatis* were noted by Bedson and Bland (1934). Localization of the inclusions to the transitional epithelium of the cervix was suggested by Thygeson and Mengert (1936). Thygeson and his co-workers also studied gynaecological patients with both gonococcal and non-gonococcal cervicitis (Thygeson and Stone, 1942). They found 5 inclusion-positive patients in each group. They also reported the investigation of 100 men with urethritis, demonstrating (by the inoculation of baboon conjunctivae) inclusions in 7 patients with gonorrhoea, and in 2 patients with NGU. Whether the patients with gonorrhoea developed PGU is not recorded. Also noted in this paper was the frequent association of inclusion conjunctivitis in babies with a history of urethritis in the father.

Despite the pioneer work described above there was still doubt, in the minds of some, of the very existence of NGU. Mast (1948), quoted by Harkness (1950), talks of penicillin-resistant gonorrhoea in a US navy ship, claiming that this was a new disease. Harkness noted that whilst inclusions were demonstrable in many cases of NGU, attempts to culture the organism from filtrates of the discharges, using the chorio-allantoic membrane of fertilized hens' eggs were unsuccessful.

The successful isolation of the trachoma agent by T'ang *et al.* in 1957 led to the rapid revival of interest in the organism. T'ang *et al.* used the yolk sac of fertilized hens' eggs for culture. This was based on the work of Cox (1938), who described a similar technique for the isolation of rickettsiae. The first isolations were performed using penicillin to protect the eggs from superinfections, but it was soon demonstrated that this adversely affected the isolation of chlamydiae. The sensitivity of *C. trachomatis* to tetracycline, and its resistance to aminoglycosides, is also noted in this original paper.

The findings of T'ang and his co-workers were soon confirmed by others, in particular Collier and Sowa (1958) from West Africa. This group demonstrated the serological relationship between the yolk sac isolates and members of the trachoma group of organisms. Further work (Collier, Duke-Elder and Jones, 1958) established that transmission of the agent from human to human caused trachoma. Intensive research into the prevention and control of trachoma followed, including attempts to prepare a vaccine. However, the availability of a culture technique also enabled workers to re-examine the role of *C. trachomatis* in the genital tract, an area which had been neglected for many years.

The first isolation of *C. trachomatis* from genital material was by Jones, Collier and Smith, (1959), who recovered the organism from the eyes of an infant with inclusion conjunctivitis and from the cervix of the mother. The group at the Institute of Ophthalmology and the London Hospital pioneered a series of important clinical studies. *C. trachomatis* was recovered from the cervix of mothers of babies with inclusion conjunctivitis and from the urethra of their fathers. Urethral isolates were obtained from men with inclusion conjunctivitis, and from men who were sexual contacts of women with inclusion conjunctivitis (Jones, 1964; Dunlop, Jones and Al-Hussaini, 1964). The yolk sac technique was also used to study men with NGU; in the UK isolates of *C. trachomatis* were obtained from 4 of 10 men (Dunlop, Harper *et al.*, 1966), and in the USA from 5 (15 per cent) of 33 men (Holt *et al.*, 1967). Furthermore, the organism was isolated from the genital tract of female sexual contacts of men with NGU; Dunlop *et al.* (1967) obtained cervical isolates from 14 (35 per cent) of 40 of these women. At about the same time Holt *et al.* (1967) recovered chlamydiae from the cervix in 6 (42 per cent) of 42 women attending a venereal diseases clinic. Thus the essential epidemiology of chlamydial genital infection — its association with NGU, its sexual transmission and its links with adult and neonatal eye disease – was firmly re-established.

Yolk sac techniques are expensive, cumbersome and liable to technical problems, including the possibility of spurious 'isolations' through cross-contamination (Harper *et al.*, 1967). Although they marked a major advance, they were not really suitable for large scale surveys. The introduction of a tissue culture procedure for the isolation of *C. trachomatis* by Gordon and Quan (1965) was a notable advance. The method involved the centrifugation of clinical specimens on to a monolayer of suitable stationary-phase cells, followed by incubation and the staining of the cells to demonstrate inclusions. Appropriate antimicrobial agents were used to control secondary infection. The relative simplicity of this procedure made it possible to examine large numbers of clinical specimens, and it was soon observed that the new technique was far more sensitive than the older yolk sac procedure. The Institute of Ophthalmology and the London Hospital group showed that cell culture could be used to obtain isolates of chlamydiae from the genital tract, rectum, eye, and other sites (Dunlop, Hare *et al.*, 1969). Again, correlation of ocular and genital infections and recovery of the agents from many men with NGU and from their female contacts were demonstrated (Dunlop, Hare *et al.*, 1971a).

A review of the isolations of *C. trachomatis* from the human genital tract was presented by Gordon and Quan at the Symposium on Trachoma and Related Disorders in Boston, in 1970 (Gordon and Quan, 1971). They reported a collaborative study involving five laboratories. Using a standard cell culture technique, the isolation rates in NGU were found to vary between 42 and 12 per cent. One factor to explain this difference could have been the different techniques of specimen collection used. The data imply that the use of an endo-urethral curette was more efficient than either a meatal cotton wool swab or bacteriological loop. Similarly, Philip, *et al.* (1971) found the urethral curette to be more efficient.

The early difficulties encountered with the culture of *C. trachomatis* in the laboratory had resulted in attempts to use serological methods. Initially, the only test available was complement fixation (CF), using a psittacosis or lymphogranuloma venereum antigen. The test was too insensitive to be of value in the investigation of superficial infections, such as inclusion conjunctivitis and NGU. The micro-immunofluorescence (micro-IF) test developed by Wang (1971) proved to be a major advance over the CF test. It became possible to introduce a serotyping scheme for strains of *C. trachomatis* (Wang and Grayston 1971). With the use of specific antigens, the test may also be used for antibody studies in serum, tears, and genital discharge. Dwyer, Treharne *et al.*, (1972) demonstrated the specificity of Wang's micro-IF test, showing its ability to differentiate *C. psittaci* from *C. trachomatis*, and also the presence of antibody to specific serotypes of the latter in sera from infected patients. The micro-IF test has however proved disappointing as a primary diagnostic test for *C. trachomatis* genital infections, except in special circumstances (see page 32); it has greater value for epidemiological surveys.

It is now clear the *ocular* strains of *C. trachomatis* are clinically and epidemiologically distinct from *genital* strains. Ocular strains cause classical trachoma: transmission is from eye to eye, and the disease has maximum prevalence in hot dry climates where standards of hygiene are low. Genital strains on the other hand are sexually transmitted and either cause or initiate many genital diseases notably, NGU, PGU and epididymitis in men and cervicitis and salpingitis in women. Ocular infection with genital strains may occur in adults by the accidental transfer of genital material to the eye, and in neonates by infection during birth. Other neonatal chlamydial infections, notably an afebrile pneumonia syndrome, have now been discovered. The immunotypes of *C. trachomatis* recovered from patients with lymphogranuloma venereum (LGV) are immunologically and biologically quite distinct from both ocular and genital strains, and LGV itself bears no clinical resemblance to other chlamydial diseases.

Genital chlamydiae are believed to cause many diseases in men, women and infants, far more than was previously thought. A list of these conditions is given in Table 1.1. The spectrum of disease associated with *C. trachomatis* has been expanding within the last few years, and further additions to the list may soon be made, but it is already clear the *C. trachomatis* is an important organism in human society.

Strenuous attempts have been made to produce a vaccine against trachoma. In spite of intensive work at a number of centres, the early hopes have not been

Table 1.1 Diseases associated with *C. trachomatis* infection

Adult disease

Trachoma
Inclusion conjunctivitis

Non-gonococcal urethritis
Post-gonococcal urethritis
Epididymitis
Proctitis

Cervicitis
Infection of Bartholin's ducts
Salpingitis
Perihepatitis

Infertility
Fetal loss
Cervical dysplasia
Urethral syndrome   } Role not yet defined
Reiter's syndrome
Bronchitis/pneumonia
Endocarditis

Fetal and neonatal disease

Inclusion conjunctivitis
Pharyngeal infection
Pneumonia
Otitis media
Vulvovaginitis

Prematurity
Low birth weight   } Role not yet defined
Gastro-intestinal infection

realised, but much useful data on the immunology of chlamydial infection has accumulated as a result of these studies. Technical problems proved an early major challenge, particularly with regard to purification of antigens, estimation of their potency, and the monitoring of field tests. The epidemiology of trachoma varies in different endemic areas, making population selection difficult. The major conclusion from vaccine studies would appear to be that modest, and frequently short-lived, protection against ocular infection challenge is possible. However, this effect may be overshadowed by a longer-lasting hypersensitivity to infection. Thus, at present there is no effective vaccine against ocular infection, and little prospect in the foreseeable future of a vaccine against either ocular or genital strains of *C. trachomatis*. Control of chlamydial diseases must therefore be directed via chemotherapeutic and epidemiological techniques.

2

Microbiology of *C. trachomatis*

Taxonomy of *C. trachomatis*

Because chlamydiae will not grow on conventional media, and because of difficulty in placing the group taxonomically, these organisms have suffered from periods of neglect and from a confused terminology. The main reason for taxonomic confusion lay in the difficulty of early workers in establishing whether the organisms were viruses or bacteria. Page (1966) extensively reviewed the morphology, cytology, chemical nature and metabolism of these organisms, and established that they were bacteria. A proliferation of intended names had preceded Page's review, for example *Miyagwanella, Ehrlichia, Chlamydozoon, Rickettsiaformis, Rakeia, Chlamydia, Bedsonia,* and *Colettsia.* Other authors used vernacular terms, such as PLV (Psittacosis-lymphogranuloma-vereneum), POMP (Psittacosis-ornithosis-mammalian pneumonitis), TRIC (Trachoma-inclusion-conjunctivitis) and PLT (Psittacosis-lymphogranuloma-trachoma). These were aptly described by Page as hyphenated monstrosities.

The early trachoma workers, Halberstaedter and von Prowazek (1907) suggested a family name *Chlamydozoa* (derived from the Greek *chlamys,* meaning a mantle, to indicate the matrix seen around the elementary bodies in Giemsa-stained preparations). Jones, Rake and Stearns (1945) amplified the differences between the rickettsiae and the chlamydiae, and gave the first taxonomically valid use of the name *Chlamydia.* Meyer in 1953 suggested that one way out of the taxonomic controversy was to use the name *Bedsonia* for the psittacosis organisms, to commemorate the work of Bedson. Whilst the suggestion was excellent on historical grounds, the priority rule gives *Chlamydia* preference (Jones, Rake and Stearns 1945).

Between 1957 (Bergey's 7th Manual of Determinative Bacteriology) and 1975 (Bergey's 8th Manual) the controversy centred around the number of genera in the family Chlamydiacae. Moulder's work (1964, 1966) divided the family into two sub-groups. Sub-group A contained the agents of trachoma and allied diseases, and sub-group B contained the psittacosis group. As a result, Page (1968) proposed two species in a single genus, namely *C. trachomatis* for sub-group A, and *C. psittaci* for sub-group B. The chlamydiae are

6

still placed in the rickettsias in Bergey's 8th manual. This appears to be largely a matter of convenience. The group is unrelated to the Rickettsiae; similarities in their life cycle probably represent convergent evolution.

Morphology and nature of *C. trachomatis*

The chlamydiae are a well defined group of prokaryotic organisms, which are characterized as small Gram negative cocci. The organisms live an obligate intracellular parasitic existence, with two distinct forms. They share a common group antigen.

The chlamydiae were originally thought to be viruses, because of their small size and their inability to survive on non-living culture media. Table 2.1 lists the characteristics of *Chlamydia* in comparison with those of bacteria, mycoplasmas and viruses.

Table 2.1 Characteristics of chlamydiae, bacteria, mycoplasmas and viruses

	Chlamydiae	Bacteria	Mycoplasmas	Viruses
Size (<500 nm)	+	−	+	+
Cell wall	+	+	−	−
DNA/RNA	+	+	+	−
Nucleoid without limiting membrane	+	+	+	−
Metabolism of carbohydrate	+	+	+	−
Ribosomes of prokaryotic type	+	+	+	−
Eclipse on infection	−	−	−	+
Incorporation with host nucleic acid	−	−	−	+
Binary fission	+	+	+	−
Inhibition by antibiotics	+	+	+	−
Growth on non-living culture media	−	+	+	−

The two distinct forms of the organism are termed the **elementary** body and the **initial** or **reticulate** body. The elementary body is the smaller particle, of around 300 nm in size. This is the extracellular transport form. It is highly infectious, and characteristically stains bluish-red with Giesma stain. The cell wall is a rigid trilaminar structure, analogous to the cell wall of Gram-negative bacteria.

The initial body is between 800 and 1200 nm in size. It is of low infectivity, and represents the intracellular reproductive form; it stains bluish with Giemsa stain. Groups of these particles form the substance of the Halberstaedter and von Prowazek Körper (HPK), first described in 1907. Lindner (1910) showed that these inclusions were conglomerates of coccoid bodies, and called them initial bodies, as they were the first to appear in the developing inclusion. Inclusions may contain a mixture of the large and small particles, plus intermediate forms which appear as the elementary body develops into the initial body. The cell wall of the initial body is thinner and more fragile than that of the elementary body, and is apparently more loosely applied to the cell membrane, a fact that may be of importance in allowing the diffusion of materials in and out of the developing inclusion. The nuclear material is less electron dense than in the elementary body.

The cell wall of the particles contain lysine and D-alanine but not diaminopimelic acid. The presence of N-acetyl muramic acid (unique to bacteria) is disputed. The cell wall of the initial body differs from that of the elementary body in that the peptidoglycans are not linked by peptide bridges. This may allow increased permeability of the initial body cell wall to adenosine triphosphate. Unlike the mycoplasmas, chlamydiae do not contain cholesterol in the cell wall. Large amounts of lipid and carbohydrates are present, but only small amounts of nucleic acids.

In contrast to the viruses, chlamydiae contain both RNA and DNA. The DNA in the elementary body is located in the nucleoid as a double stranded twisted circle. The guanine-cytosine ratio is approximately 45 per cent in *C. trachomatis* (40 per cent in *C. psittaci*), and the genome size around 9.8×10^8 dalton. This is of the same order as *Mycoplasma hominis*, which is capable of independent existence. (For comparison, *Escherichia coli* has a genome size of 28×10^8 dalton, and the vaccinia virus 1.9×10^8 dalton).

As in bacterial cells, 70S ribosomes are found, divisible into 30S and 50S components. At least 18 amino acids have been described, occupying 60 per cent of the elementary body. An important point of difference from the viruses is shown by the effect of cycloheximide (Tribby, Friis and Moulder, 1973). This compound inhibits the ribosomal synthesis of eukaryotic but not prokaryotic cells. Chlamydiae are not affected by this compound, showing that unlike viruses they do not make use of the host cell translation apparatus, but synthesize their own DNA protein.

The chlamydiae are primarily energy parasites, acquiring ATP from the host cell. However, it has been shown (Weiss *et al.*, 1964) that anaerobic metabolism of glucose does occur, probably via the pentose phosphate pathway, and one of the glyoclytic pathways. This activity is at a low level and under abnormal conditions it appears to produce a net *loss* of ATP and NAD. Electron transport systems are apparently absent, although both particles contain cyto-chrome C reductase. Host cell macromolecular synthesis is somehow shut down by the chlamydiae, and the host cell high energy substances diverted to the synthesis of chlamydial proteins and lipids. The host cell provides metabolites also, which are derived from its pool rather than by degradation. Some of these metabolites (eg isoleucine) may be inhibitory to chlamydial growth, and hence possibly involved in latency of chlamydial infections (Hatch, 1975).

Chlamydiae are highly adapted to their intracellular life. They may well have derived from other bacteria which led an increasingly intracellular existence, overcoming the efforts of the host cell phagocytic systems to destroy them. Certainly the almost total absence of biochemical mechanisms for producing energy would alone restrict them to an intracellular existence.

Life-cycle of *C. trachomatis*

Entry of the elementary body into the host cell is by phagocytosis; there is no evidence of an ATP utilizing active transport system as is found in the Rickettsiae. Chlamydiae are in some way able specifically to induce their own phagocytosis, which is of obvious advantage to an obligate intracellular parasite. Ingestion of the elementary body is accompanied by its uncoating, with resultant softening of the cell wall. The presence of the infective particle within the phagosome is not accompanied by fusion with lysosomes, as in the normal process of phagocytosis. This phenomenon is directed by the chlamydiae, as is demonstrated by the observation that following the ingestion of heat-killed chlamydiae lysosome fusion does occur (Friis, 1972). Further, non-professional (ie not actively phagocytozing) cells, are specifically induced by the chlamydiae to ingest them (Byrne and Moulder 1978).

The elementary body lies therefore in a vacuole surrounded by a host cell derived membrane, protected from the action of lysozyme. Unlike viruses, chlamydiae have no eclipse phase. Without loss of individuality, the elementary body enlarges to form the metabolically active initial body. During this phase, there is active production of RNA by the particle. The mRNA is produced on the DNA chromosome using a DNA-dependant RNA polymerase contained within the elementary body. Ribosomal and tRNA are also found in the elementary body. This process takes seven to ten hours, during which time the phagosome moves centripetally to the host cell nucleus. The initial body thus formed begins to undergo binary fission to form further initial bodies. The generation time is two to three hours. The method of binary fission is still controversial. Moulder (1966) believed that the majority of evidence favoured cross wall formation, as electron dense bridges had been demonstrated between large cells that had apparently just completed division. Moulder also quoted evidence for structures possibly similar to the mesosomes of true bacteria. Work by Armstrong and Reed (1967) suggested that circumferential constrictions leading to fission occurred. Still further controversy surrounds the possibility of multiple endosporulation as an alternative mechanism (Kramer and Gordon, 1971). This latter, if it occurs at all, is at such low frequency that it is unlikely to be quantitatively important. With increasing numbers of initial bodies, the inclusions enlarge to form the characteristic semilunar mantle around the host cell nucleus (Fig 2.1). At this stage, *C. trachomatis* (but not *C. psittaci*) lays down a glycogen matrix, responsible for the brown staining of the inclusions with iodine. After ten to fifteen hours, DNA again becomes detectable. This corresponds to condensation of the initial bodies from 800 nm to 300 nm, to produce elementary bodies. Intermediate

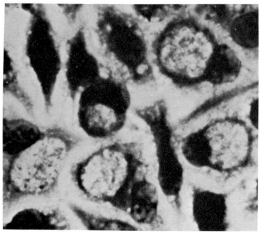

Fig. 2.1   Mature inclusions of *C. trachomatis* in IUDR-treated McCoy cells. (Giemsa-stained)

stages are seen, with increasingly electron dense regions as the nucleoid reforms. Gradually, all the initial bodies are replaced by elementary bodies, so that thirty-six to forty-eight hours after infection the mature inclusions are ready to release the infectious elementary bodies. Rupture of the host cell occurs, following a sequential process of damage to the host cell membrane, and the chlamydial growth cycle is completed.

Serology of *C. trachomatis*

The chlamydiae (*C. trachomatis* and *C. psittaci*) share a common group reactive complement fixing (CF) antigen. This antigen is an acidic polysaccharide of high molecular weight (Grayston and Wang, 1975). Whilst of use for the serodiagnosis of psittacosis and lymphogranuloma vereneum, the CF test has proved too insensitive for the diagnosis of oculo-genital infections with *C. trachomatis*. The development of the micro-IF test by Wang (1971) allowed the separation of *C. trachomatis* into fifteen serotypes (Grayson and Wang, 1975). The serological inter-relationships of these serotypes are complex, and the antigens have not been identified biochemically. In Table 2.2 the serotypes are arranged in relationship to the diseases they tend to produce. Type A is largely restricted to the Middle East and North Africa, and Ba to trachoma among North American Indians. These strains are almost exclusive to hyperendemic trachoma. D and E are the serotypes most commonly associated with genital infection, and with inclusion conjunctivitis of adults (paratrachoma), and neonates (inclusion blennorrhoea). Even in countries where trachoma is hyperendemic, genital infection tends to be with serotypes D and E. Serotypes G and F are the next most frequently isolated. In non-endemic areas, ocular strains isolated show a similar serotypic distribution to the genital strains isolated, irrespective of whether the ocular disease is trachoma, paratrachoma, or inclusion conjunctivitis of neonates. L1 and L2 cross react widely with other serotypes, and may be used in single antigen tests for the presence of chlamydial antibody in human serum (Thomas, Reeve and Oriel, 1976) (*see* page 115).

The host serological response to chlamydial infection, as demonstrated by micro-IF testing, is complex. Serum antibodies of IgG or IgM, and local (tear or cervical) antibodies of IgG or IgA class, are produced. However, it is becoming apparent that among the sexually promiscuous background levels of antibody are high (Schachter, 1978). Further, IgM antibodies may be short-lived. There is also evidence that the serological response to subsequent re-infection may be directed initially against earlier serotypes (Wang and Grayston, 1971, *see* page 21). The predictive value of serum antibody thus

Table 2.2   Serotypes of *Chlamydia trachomatis*

Hyperendemic trachoma	A	B	Ba	C	J		
Genital infection and paratrachoma	D	E	F	G	H	I	K
Lymphogranuloma venereum	L_1	L_2	L_3				

relies heavily on the timing of several specimens. The best results have been with the detection of IgM or seroconversion in males with first attack urethritis (Bowie, Alexander and Holmes, 1977). It is possible that the detection of IgM antibody will be useful in the diagnosis of chlamydial infections in neonates, particularly the pneumonitis syndrome.

Tear antibodies are found in both trachoma and inclusion conjunctivitis (Grayston and Wang, 1975). More recently McComb, *et al.* (1979) examined cervical secretion antibodies and concluded that these antibodies were of more useful predictive value for current infection with *C. trachomatis*, than were serum antibodies. In contrast, Schachter, Cles *et al.* (1979a) and Richmond, Paul and Taylor, (1980) concluded that neither serum or cervical antibodies were useful in predicting active infection.

Attempts to simplify the micro-IF test currently being reported from a number of centres (*see* page 31) are designed not only to ease the technical demands of the test, but also to improve the diagnostic value in relation to current infection. We are still a long way from understanding the host response to both local and systemic infection with *C. trachomatis*.

The antimicrobial sensitivities of *C. trachomatis*

Methods of investigation

The sensitivity of *C. trachomatis* to various antimicrobials has proved useful in elucidating its microbiological characteristics, and providing guidelines for treatment. However, the methods used in the past for in-vitro studies have been cumbersome, and often produced discrepant results between different workers. Jawetz (1969) extensively reviewed the chemotherapy of chlamydial infections, and attributed these discrepancies to the large number of variables within and between the methods used. He concluded that most weight must be placed on adequately controlled therapeutic studies in natural hosts. At that time, such studies were regrettably few, and frequently anecdotal. Over the last ten years, the major advances in culture techniques have led to a greater understanding of the action of antimicrobial agents on *C. trachomatis*.

Following the description by T'ang *et al.*, (1957) of the use of the yolk sac of embryonated hen's eggs to culture *C. trachomatis*, the method was adapted to investigate the action of antimicrobial agents on chlamydiae. One of the most extensive reports was by Werner (1961), who studied the effects of a wide range of antimicrobials in yolk sac culture. The percentage of eggs protected was plotted against the logarithmic dose of antimicrobial agent used. From these data, a minimal effective dose for each antimicrobial was calculated. Gordon and Quan (1962) assayed the antimicrobial effect by calculation of the logarithmic titre of inclusions in killed eggs protected with the antimicrobial agent under test, against the logarithmic titre of inclusions in unprotected eggs. Werner's experiments were concerned with antimicrobials of possible therapeutic use (i.e. penicillins, tetracyclines, sulphonamides and macrolides), whilst Gordon and Quan were attempting to improve the isolation of *Chlamydia* in yolk sac (and later in tissue culture) by the protection of the culture system from microbial contamination, using antimicrobial agents with no antichlamydial activity (e.g. streptomycin, bacitracin, nystatin, and polymixin B). Percentage protection was also used by Sowa and Race (1971) in a study on the aminoglycosides for isolation purposes. Other workers calculated the protective dose$_{50}$ (Johnson, 1962), or logarithmic 'virus' inactivation (Jawetz, 1962), as indices of antimicrobial activity.

In an attempt to standardize laboratory procedure, Tarizzo and Nabli (1967) demonstrated a linear relationship between the egg lethal dose$_{50}$ (ELD$_{50}$) and the average day of death of the embryonated eggs. This relationship obviated the need for infectivitiy titrations, allowing the use of single dilution controls — a considerable saving of time and materials. These workers investigated not only therapeutic agents (tetracycline and erythromycin), but also a wide range of antiseptics (Nabli and Tarizzo, 1967). Alcohols, chlorine, iodine, formalin, acids and bases inactivated chlamydiae after 1–30 min of contact. Shiao, Wang and Grayston (1967) described strains of *C. trachomatis* showing decreased sensitivity to tetracyclines, penicillins and to sulphonamides. The assay method involved the demonstration of a reduction in the egg infective dose$_{50}$ (EID$_{50}$).

Differences between the results of various workers led Ghione *et al.* (1967) to study the peculiarities of the hen's egg as an experimental model. They concluded that the results could be affected by the ability of the egg to take up or metabolize the antimicrobial agent, reducing the amount available to act against the infecting organism.

Reeve *et al.* (1968) investigated the action of the folic acid inhibitors on *C. trachomatis* using an egg culture system. Percentage survival of eggs was calculated, and the increase in mean survival time. A constant dose of infecting agent was used (10^{6}ELD$_{50}$), and the increase in mean survival time plotted against the logarithmic dose of antimicrobial agent to give a regression line. This technique proved convenient and reproducible, and was later used to examine other antimicrobial agents (Reeve, 1976; Ridgway, 1982). The results of these experiments confirmed the *in vitro* efficacy of the tetracyclines and erthromycin, and the partial efficacy of sulphonamides and penicillins. Trimethoprim and the aminoglycosides were shown to have little antichlamydial activity. The possible therapeutic effect of rifampicin against *C. trachomatis* was also initially demonstrated in egg culture, by Becker and Zackay-Rones (1969).

In ovo methods involve the use of high infective doses of *Chlamydia*. An increase in mean survival time of one day represents the inactivation of $10^6 ELD_{50}$. Large numbers of eggs are required for each experiment, and must be tended for up to thirteen days. Unpredictable early deaths of the eggs occur, and a premature end to the study may be precipitated by hatching. The inefectivity of eggs is known to show a seasonal variation (Jawetz, 1969), and thermal inactivation of the antimicrobial agent may occur (Treharne *et al.*, 1977). Many of the experiments described used high concentrations of antimicrobial agents, levels which if attainable in humans may prove toxic. *In vitro* activity in the egg culture system may thus bear little relationship to therapeutic usefulness. The criteria used to evaluate egg culture studies have differed widely, so it is difficult to interpret the significance of individual results or to compare results between investigators.

Mice have been used as an alternative to eggs. The major problem with this animal is the establishment of infection. Werner (1961) used the intracerebral route of inoculation, and administered antimicrobial agents either orally or subcutaneously. Percentage protection, based on survival time, was used to evaluate antimicrobial activity. The subjectivity of mouse experiments was well summarized by Jawetz (1969). He noted that mice could be infected intracerebrally or intraperitoneally, and could receive the antimicrobial prophylactically or therapeutically, in single or multiple dosage. 'The earlier a drug is administered and the longer high levels are maintained, the greater the likelihood of survival of the animal, or even the eradication of the infecting agent. The later drug administration is started, the greater the probability of persistent infection in surviving animals'. Primates have also been used to evaluate antimicrobial activity in chlamydial conjunctivitis, but with limited success.

The successful culture of *C. trachomatis* in eggs was followed by the adaptation of isolates to cell culture. Initially, cells derived from developing chicks were used, such as the entodermal culture of Gordon and Quan (1962). Bernkopf, Mashiah and Becker (1962) were able to adapt one of T'ang's original strains to grow in fetal lung cells. Both the above workers used reduction in inclusion count to measure antimicrobial activity. As was the practice with egg experiments, cell cultures were protected by antimicrobials in addition to the antimicrobial under test, which could arguably invalidate the results.

An advantage of cell culture for investigating antimicrobial activity is the ability to observe the action under the microscope. Armstrong and Reed (1967) described the appearance of inclusions treated with penicillin, experiments useful in elucidating the taxonomic position of these organisms.

Ridgway, Owen and Oriel (1976) described a simplified, standardizable technique for the investigation of antimicrobial activity, using idoxuridine treated McCoy cells. Doubling dilutions of antimicrobial were added to antimicrobial-free growth medium, which was then inoculated with a reference strain of *C. trachomatis*. Following incubation, cell monolayers were fixed, and stained with Giemsa or iodine stain, and examined under the light microscope for the presence or absence of inclusions. A minimum inhibitory concentration (MIC) could thus be determined. The method was suitable for the investigation of clinical isolates, and by the use of multiple passage could be extended to give a minimum bactericidal concentration(MBC). As had been reported by other workers, it was found that most antimicrobials gave a definite end-point, with the notable exception of the penicillins, cephalosporins and the folic acid inhibitors. Other similar techniques have been described (Treharne, Day, *et al.*, 1977; Kuo, Wang and Grayston, 1978; and Lee, Bowie and Alexander, 1978). The numerical values of the results, and the details of the methods vary, but the order of activity against *C. trachomatis* of the various antimicrobials examined is in agreement. An important difference in methodology in these more recent studies from the early experiments was that antimicrobial agents were not used to prevent the contamination of cultures. Bowie, Lee and Alexander (1978) examined a number of variations in technique, particularly the timing of the addition of the antimicrobial agents in relation to inoculation of the cell culture. This factor has been the subject of some controversy. They found a better correlation with clinical studies on chronic trachoma when antimicrobial agents were added after forty-eight hours of incubation; addition of antimicrobial agents earlier in the growth cycle correlated well with clinical studies on genital chlamydial infections, a finding in agreement with the workers noted above.

Sensitivity of *C. trachomatis* to antimicrobial agents

Antimicrobial agents showing good in-vitro activity against *C. trachomatis* are shown in Table 2.3. In this group are the tetracyclines, the macrolides, and rifampicin. Rifampicin is the most active compound tested against chlamydiae, but as is common with other bacteria the development of in-vitro resistance to rifamycins may be readily demonstrated (Ridgway, Boulding and Lam Po Tang, 1979). There is cross resistance between rifampicin and rifamide. All the tetracyclines tested and the various salts of erythromycin have essentially the same in-vitro activity. Rosaramicin, a new macrolide, is more active than erythromycin.

Table 2.4 shows antimicrobial agents with no useful activity against *C. trachomatis*. The aminoglycosides and vancomycin are useful in protecting cultures from contamination. The lack of activity of metronidazole is consistent with the poor response seen in the therapy of NGU with this compound. Spectinomycin, cefuroxime and trimethoprim (in cotrimoxazole) all have a place in the treatment of gonorrhoea, but these agents are not effective against concurrent chlamydial infection.

The antimicrobials shown in Table 2.5 have demonstrable activity against *C. trachomatis*, as seen by the MIC results. However they are disappointing when used to treat chlamydial infections. If a cell culture is treated with increasing concentrations of a penicillin, the morphology of the inclusions changes to give the globular effect shown in Fig 2.2 (in comparison with the normal inclusion in antimicrobial-free medium shown in Fig 2.3) (Johnson and Hobson 1977). Higher concentrations of penicillin result in inclusions that are empty, or can no longer be seen. However, replacement of the penicillin-

Table 2.3 Minimum inhibitory concentrations (MIC) of various antimicrobial agents with high activity against *C. trachomatis* in cell culture

Antimicrobial agents	MIC mg/l
Rifampicin	0.007
Rosaramicin	0.015
Doxycycline	0.03
Minocycline	0.03
Oxytetracycline	0.06
Erythromycin	0.06

Table 2.4 Minimum inhibitory concentrations (MIC) of various antimicrobial agents with low activity against *C. trachomatis* in cell culture

Antimicrobial agents	MIC mg/l
Spectinomycin	64
Oxolinic acid	128
Trimethoprim	128
Cefuroxime	256
Lincomycin	512
Vancomycin	>256
Metronidazole	>256
Gentamicin	>512
Cefotaxime	>512

Table 2.5 Minimum inhibitory concentrations (MIC) of various antimicrobial agents with medium activity against *C. trachomatis* in cell culture

Antimicrobial	MIC mg/l
Ampicillin	0.25
Mecillinam	0.25
Thiamphenicol	0.5
Penicillin	1.0
Clindamycin	1.0
Rifamide	1.0
Amoxycillin	2.0
Cephaloridine	2.0
Sulphamethoxazole	4.0
Chloramphenicol	4.0
Fusidic Acid	4.0
Tioconazole	16.0

containing medium with antimicrobial-free medium will result in recovery of these inclusions, albeit usually after multiple passage on to fresh host cells (Table 2.6). Similarly, the tiny inclusions produced with the folic acid inhibitors may revert to normal after antimicrobial-free passage (Fig. 2.4, Fig. 2.5). Chloramphenicol and thiamphenicol do not produce gross morphological changes in the inclusions as seen with the light microscope, but again multiple

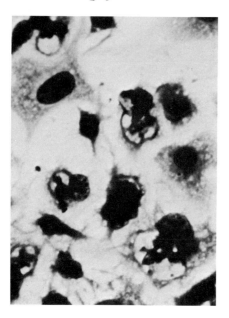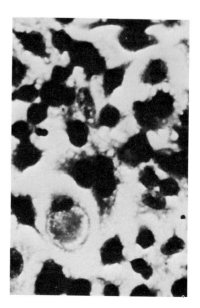

Fig 2.2   Abnormal inclusions of *C. trachomatis* induced by penicillin. (IUDR-treated McCoy cells, Giemsa stained)

Fig 2.3   Normal inclusions of *C. trachomatis* in antimicrobial-free medium (URDR-treated McCoy cells, Giemsa-stained)

Table 2.6   Effect of passage on growth of *C. trachomatis* after initial incubation with cephaloridine

Cephaloridine mg/l in first tube	Passage			
	0	1	2	3
0.5	+*	+	+	+
1.0	+	+	+	+
2.0	−	+	+	+
4.0	−	+	+	+
8.0	−	−	+	+
16.0	−	−	−	+
32.0	−	−	−	+

+* = Iodine stained inclusions present
MIC for cephaloridine = 2 mg/l
MBC for cephaloridine = >32 mg/l

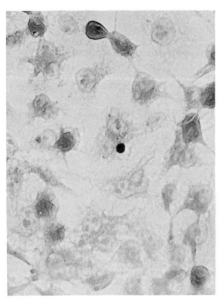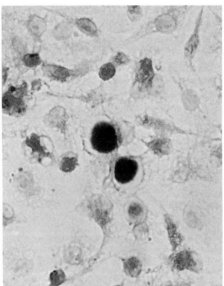

Fig. 2.4 Abnormal inclusions of *C. trachomatis* induced by sulphonamide. (IUDR-treated McCoy cells, iodine stained)

Fig. 2.5 Normal inclusions of *C. trachomatis* in antimicrobial-free medium. (IUDR-treated McCoy cells, iodine stained)

Table 2.7 Effect of passage on growth of *C. trachomatis* after initial incubation with thiamphenicol

Thiamphenicol mg/l	Passage number						
	0	1	2	3	4	5	6
0.015	+						
0.03	+						
0.06	+						
0.12	+						
0.25	+	+					
0.5	−	+	+				
1.0	−	−	+	+			
2.0	−	−	−	+	+		
4.0	−	−	−	−	−	+	
8.0	−	−	−	−	−	−	+

MIC for thiamphenicol = 0.5 mg/l
MBC for thiamphenicol = > 8.0 mg/l

passage will produce an MBC much higher than would be found after single passage (Table 2.7). It is possible that these antimicrobial agents induce a form of latency in *C. trachomatis* (see page 19). This could explain the clinical finding that when the agents listed in Table 2.5 are used to treat chlamydial infection, apparent cure may be followed later by relapse with re-isolation of *C.*

Table 2.8 Relationship between MIC and MBC for *C. trachomatis* against various antimicrobials (after Ridgway, Owen and Oriel (1978) and Ridgway and Oriel (1979)

	MIC (mg/l)	MBC (mg/l)	Number of passages to end-point
Rifampicin	0.007	0.06	2
Rosaramicin	0.015	0.06	2
Minocycline	0.03	0.25	2
Oxytetracycline	0.06	0.25	2
Erythromycin	0.06	0.5	3
Mecillinam	0.25	>1.0	2
Thiamphenicol	0.5	>8.0	6
Cephaloridine	2.0	>32	3
Fusidic acid	4.0	64	3
Chloramphenicol	4.0	16	3
Sulphamethoxazole	4.0	32	6
Spectinomycin	64	128	1
Trimethoprim	128	1024	3
Cefuroxime	256	512	1

trachomatis. Most antimicrobial agents examined by this technique induce latency to some extent, although the tetracyclines and the macrolides still have a clinically useful MBC. It is clear therefore that the MIC is an unreliable means of predicting anti-chlamydial activity, as is a single passage MBC. Table 2.8 gives the relationship between the MIC and the MBC of various antimicrobial agents.

The MIC of related antimicrobial agents, for example rifampicin and rifamide, clindamycin and linomycin, and the penicillins and cephalosporins, may differ markedly (*see* Table 2.3–2.5). It is not therefore possible to predict the activity of other members of an antimicrobial group from the results obtained for one member. The reasons for these discrepancies are not clear, but may be related to the ability of a drug to enter the host cell. There is almost no data on the intracellular concentrations of antimicrobial agents.

Antimicrobial agents also have different effects on the staining properties of chlamydial inclusions. Penicillins inhibit glycogen production (Jawetz, 1969), which may result in the failure of iodine staining. Folic acid inhibitors prevent autofluorescence, but iodine stained inclusions may still be present. In consequence, experiments must utilize both staining methods to give valid results.

Jawetz (1969) summarized the advantages and disadvantages of cell culture systems. He drew attention to the single cycle of growth produced *in vitro*, to the differing suscpetibility of cell lines, and to the necessity for an arbitrary end point, e.g. formation of inclusions, release of infective particles etc. In spite of these disadvantages, it remains likely that the study of drug activity in cell culture will reveal information applicable to therapeutic problems. It is impossible at present to devise an in-vitro technique which will accurately mimic the asynchronous intracellular infection seen clinically. The intrinsic anti-chlamydial activity of the host cell cannot be controlled, and the role of host defences in conjunction with the antimicrobial agents both in cell culture and in clinical infection is unknown. Too much discussion has been expended in an attempt to extrapolate numerical values of MICs and MBCs to the clinical situation. The cell culture results give no more than an indication of clinical activity, and the final arbiter remains the controlled clinical trial.

Latency in *C. trachomatis* infections

A fundamental biological characteristic of chlamydial infection is the production of latent, persistent, and inapparent infections (Manire, 1977). Meyer and Eddie (1951) recorded chronic inapparent infection in a patient who acquired psittacosis in 1938. Upon recovery, he continued to shed organisms for the next eight years, until intensive penicillin therapy terminated his carrier state. During this period, his only symptoms were an occasional cough with tenacious sputum. Inapparent infections in flocks of domestic birds may only be revealed following outbreaks of disease in poultry workers (Irons, Sullivan and Rowen, 1951).

A number of in-vitro models for latency have been described, using *C. psittaci*. Manire and Galasso (1959) were able to establish latent infection of HeLa cells with a meningo-pneumonitis agent. Addition of penicillin to the cultures suppressed production of infectious particles, but on its removal, regular production of elementary bodies soon commenced. This finding is of particular interest in relation to the antimicrobial experiments described earlier (see page 14). Hatch (1975) described an experimental model of *C. psittaci* infection, which showed that multiplication could be inhibited by a reduction in the availability of isoleucine in the immediate environment of the inclusion. The inclusions remain viable, and the latent infection could be re-activated by treatment of the host cells with cycloheximide (thus reducing host cell macromolecular synthesis).

Hanna, Dawson *et al.* (1968) used direct immunofluorescent staining of conjunctival cells to demonstrate persistent infection in the conjunctivae of patients without current clinical activity of trachoma or inclusion conjunctivitis. These findings were supported by experiments in volunteers, and the authors concluded that latent ocular infection with *C. trachomatis* was common. Gale, Wang and Grayston, (1971) reported the persistence of ocular infection in two Taiwan monkeys for over ten years. Whether these infections indicate latency or merely a chronic inapparent disease is a matter of opinion.

The relevance of these findings to genital infections is unknown. Schachter and Dawson (1978) note that it is not inconsistent for chlamydiae to act either as primary pathogens, or as causes of inapparent infection in the same host species. Schachter (1978) states that it would be wrong to assume that chlamydiae are part of the normal flora when found in the clinically inapparent state, and he suggests that latent or sub-clinical infections represent an interaction between the host cell defence mechanisms, and persistent low levels of chlamydial multiplication. To what extent latency is a feature of genital chlamydial infection remains conjectural, along with the consequences of such infection, if it exists.

Animal models of C. trachomatis infection

A major stumbling block to research into the pathogenicity of *C. trachomatis* is the lack of a suitable animal model. The only animals with any useful susceptibility are the expensive non-human primates. Even here, the susceptibility of different species varies. For example, chimpanzees (*Pan* spp.) and baboons (*Papio* spp.) are more susceptible than macaques (*Macaca* spp.), particularly to genital infections.

Primates are not only expensive but inconvenient to handle, and attempts have therefore been made to use other animals. The chlamydial strains mostly used belong to *C. psittaci*, simply because these strains are endemic in non-primates. Since there are important biological differences between *C. trachomatis* and *C. psittaci*, the relevance of experiments with the latter organisms to human disease must be in doubt, although much useful information has been obtained. Mount *et al.*, (1973) infected male guinea-pig urethras, using a guinea-pig inclusion conjunctivitis strain (GPIC), and demonstrated transmission to females. Darougar *et al.*, (1977) again using the GPIC agent noted similarities to chlamydial conjunctivitis in humans, but were unable to reproduce the pannus and scarring characteristic of trachoma. However they noted that recurrent infection results in a shortened but more severe form of conjunctivitis, with a change in the inflammatory response from predominantly polymorphonuclear to lymphocytic. They were able to produce blindness in the cat by repeated inoculation of a feline strain of *C. psittaci* in conjunction with other bacteria (e.g. normal throat flora). This would suggest that another factor in the pathogenesis of chlamydial disease may be the combined action of chlamydiae and other bacteria. The cat strain is of particular interest, as it naturally affects the genital tract also. Recently, Howard, O'Leary and Nichols (1976) have demonstrated immunity of guinea-pigs to subsequent re-infection with GPIC agent. It is noteworthy that the eyes were still susceptible after urethral infection, but that neither eyes nor urethra could be re-infected after ocular infection. Localization of the GPIC agent to the squamo-columnar junction of the cervix of guinea-pigs was demonstrated by Barron *et al.*, (1979). The inclusions were restricted to the columnar cells of this region, and not found in the true endocervical columnar cells. This may provide a useful model for studying cervical infection.

Studies of infection of non-human primates with *C. trachomatis* antedated its isolation. Lindner (1909) produced a disease similar to inclusion conjunctivitis in a macaque and a baboon, using cervical secretions from the mother of a child with inclusion blennorrhoea. Darougar, Kinnison and Jones (1971) infected the eyes of two baboons, and the urethra of a third with a strain of *C. trachomatis* isolated from the rectum of the mother of a neonate with chlamydial inclusion conjunctivitis. The literature is in general inconclusive on the production of a urethral discharge in non-human primates. Digiacomo, *et al.*, (1975) succeeded with some difficulty in infecting the urethras of two baboons with a serotype D *C. trachomatis*. They were able to follow the infection serologically using the micro-IF test (*see* page 30). One baboon required two attempts to produce infection. After infection had been established the animals excreted the organism for 90 and 96 days respectively. A specific antibody response was obtained. Subsequent re-inoculation of one baboon with the same strain failed to produce a marked antibody response, except for a transient rise in micro-IF titre at 14 days after the third inoculation, which disappeared within a further 14 days. The other baboon was subsequently re-inoculated with a serotype I strain on two occasions. No organisms were recovered from the first re-inoculation, and a low titre from the second. There was no antibody boost to the D serotype, and antibody directed agaist the I serotype was not detected. Further, at no time did either baboon develop a urethral discharge. The authors comment that homologous or heterologous re-infection did not significantly alter the antibody titres or the type specific response. In a later experiment (Gale *et al.*, 1977) the urethras of two out of four male pig-tailed macaques were successfully infected with an E serotype. These two monkeys yielded a low titre of *C. trachomatis* for between 40 and 55 days post infection. All four monkeys developed a type specific micro-IF titre of between 16 and 64. Urethral follicles were demonstrated in the two monkeys excreting *C. trachomatis*, but not in the others. Wang and Grayston (1971) had earlier infected eyes and cervices of Taiwan monkeys (*M. cyclopis*) with *C. trachomatis*. Re-infection of the eyes of these animals (irrespective of whether the cervix or eyes had received the primary inoculation), with a heterologous strain led to rapid recall of type specific antibody to the primary strain, followed by development of type specific anbibody to the re-infecting strain. Although these results are somewhat at variance with the findings of Digiacomo, *et al.* (1975), they indicate the possibility that serological response to a current infection may not be type specific, which may have relevance to human infections. Indeed, in patients who have had multiple *C. trachomatis* infections, with different serotypes, a single type specific antibody response may not occur.

The use of chimpanzees (*Pan* spp.) as experimental animals was reported by Jacobs, Arum and Kraus (1978). Three male animals were successfully infected intra-urethrally with a relatively low titre of infectious agent. Two of the animals developed a urethral discharge containing a moderate number of polymorphonuclear leucocytes. The progress of the infections was followed by isolation and serological (CF group antibodies) techniques. All three monkeys yielded *C. trachomatis* for between 5 and 9 weeks after infection. A four-fold rise in CF titre was demonstrated in two of the animals, and a two-fold rise in the third. Subsequently, the three chimpanzees were challenged with increasing inocula of *C. trachomatis* in the oropharynx. Two of the animals developed oropharyngeal infection with low titre shedding of *C. trachomatis*. The authors observed that whilst infection of the pharynx required higher titres of organism than infection of the urethra, they noted that they were unable to determine the influence of one chlamydial infection on another at a different site in the same animals. The same serotype (F) was used for pharyngeal and urethral experiments.

Infection of the genital tract of female monkeys has also been successfully accomplished.Braley (1939) infected the cervix of three baboons, as evidenced by experimental transmission to the conjunctivae of the same animal. Thygeson and Mengert (1936) had earlier attempted to infect a baboon's cervix, but succeeded only in demonstrating an inclusion negative cervicitis. Darougar, *et al.*, (1977) were also unable to produce cervicitis in two baboons inoculated with a D and G serotype respectively. Infection of the cervix of pregnant Taiwan monkeys (*Macaca cyclops*) by Alexander and Chiang (1967) failed to produce disease in the mother or offspring. However, ocular challenge of the infants with the same strain at 6 months produced severe disease, with pannus.

More recently, interest in the broad spectrum of chlamydial disease in man led Ripa *et al.* (1979) to demonstrate chlamydial salpingitis in grivet monkeys (*Cercopethecus aethiops*). Two monkeys were infected with a serotype K, one directly into the fallopian tubes, and the other via the cervix into the uterus. A third monkey was inoculated with serotype I into the fallopian tubes, and a fourth monkey received similarly *Chlamydia*-free medium to act as a control. Clinical salpingitis was produced in all three infected monkeys after 7 days. A purulent exudate was not produced, although the tubes were swollen and reddened with a watery exudate. *C. trachomatis* was re-isolated from all three monkeys, and a four-fold rise to both IgM and IgG by micro-IF was demonstrated. The disease was self-limiting after about 5 weeks.

Whilst these experiments with non-human primates are contributing to our knowledge of chlamydial diseases, the expense and inconvenience of handling non-human primates (as well as the valid pleas of the conservationists) means that progress using these animals as models will be restricted. There remains a need for a non-primate animal model for *C. trachomatis*. Possibly some of the difficulty in infecting animals experimentally is due to a lack of understanding of other factors in the pathogenesis, as typified by the cat experiments of Darougar, *et al.* (1977).

3

Laboratory diagnosis of *C. trachomatis*

Specimen collection

The reliable identification of *C. trachomatis* from clinical material requires close co-operation between the clinical department and the microbiology laboratory. Specimens must be carefully taken, and transported under optimal conditions. In the laboratory, a high standard of technical expertize is required both for culture and serological techniques. Failure of clinical and micro-biological procedures may lead to the return of misleading results by the laboratory.

Ideally, delay between obtaining specimens for culture and inoculation of the culture system should be minimal. In the UK, it is unlikely that a comprehensive laboratory service will be widely available in the foreseeable future, hence some form of transport system will be required (see page 114).

Urethra Specimens from the male urethra are collected using a cotton wool or calcium alginate tipped wire swab. The swab is passed approximately 4 cm into the urethra, rotated and withdrawn (Fig. 3.1). The distal 2 cm of the swab is cut off, using wire cutters, into a chlamydial transport medium (Fig. 3.2). An alternative method, using a urethral curette to scrape the wall of the urethra under local anaesthesia, offers no advantage over the swab (Dunlop, Vaughan-Jackson and Darougar, 1972).

Specimens from the female urethra are obtained as above, inserting the swab 1–2 cm into the urethra.

Cervix The site of chlamydial growth is the squamo-columnar junction of the endocervical canal. Good exposure of the cervix is essential, so the patient should be examined in the lithotomy position,and a bivalve speculum used. The cervix is cleaned with a sterile gauze swab. A cotton wool or alginate tipped swab is inserted into the cervical canal, and rotated. After withdrawal, the distal 2 cm of the swab is broken off into the transport medium.

Eyes The lower tarsal conjunctiva is sampled for the diagnosis of neonatal and adult inclusion conjunctivitis. Purulent exudate should be removed with a sterile swab, and may be examined for gonococci and other pathogens. A dry cotton wool or alginate tipped swab is then firmly rubbed across the lower

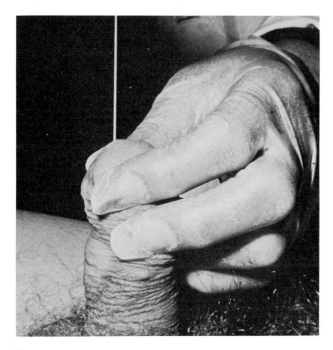

Fig. 3.1   Collection of endo-urethral specimen for chlamydial culture

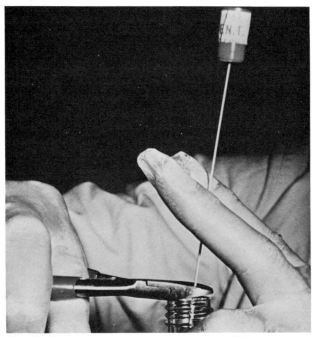

Fig. 3.2   Transfer of endo-urethral swab to chlamydial transport medium

tarsal conjunctiva. Since the inclusions will be in epithelial cells, not pus cells, it is important that the former are obtained. If direct microscopical examination is to be performed, the swab is first rubbed across a sterile glass microscope slide, and is then broken off into chlamydial transport medium.

Respiratory tract Nasopharyngeal specimens are best obtained by suction (No. 5 French gauge infant feeding tube). Alternatively, a flexible wire mounted swab may be used pernasally (Harrison, *et al.*, 1978).

Transport of specimens to the laboratory should be within twenty-four hours, during which time specimens are held at +4°C (e.g. on crushed ice). Where longer delay will be encountered, specimens should be held at −70°C, using cryo-protective medium, such as the sucrose phosphate medium recommended by Dunlop, Vaughan-Jackson and Darougar (1972).

Cytological techniques

Until the successful isolation of *C. trachomatis* in the fertilized hens' egg yolk sac, the only means of identifying the organism was by the direct microscopy of clinical material. However, the sensitivity of direct cytology in the genital tract is low. The growth of *C. trachomatis* in living culture systems (yolk sac or cell culture) also requies cytological techniques for demonstration of the organism. Stains used will either stain the developing elements within the inclusion (e.g. Giemsa), or the supporting matrix of the inclusion (e.g. iodine). The most convenient stains available for both clinical and laboratory use are Lugol's iodine, or Giemsa stain. Many other staining techniques have been described, but are more applicable to the staining of cell cultures than to the direct cytological examination of clinical specimens.

All cytological techniques for identification of *C. trachomatis* depend on the demonstration of the characteristic crescent-shaped intracytoplasmic inclusions. In suitable material, these are pathognomonic for *C. trachomatis*. However, artefacts occur, particularly after staining with Giemsa or Lugol's iodine. Considerable interpretative expertise is required if false-positive results are to be avoided. Similarly, small numbers of inclusions are easily missed by an inexperienced observer. In general, material from eyes will contain large numbers of inclusions, and it is in this field (particularly adult and neonatal conjunctivitis) that cytology is most useful for diagnosis.

The technique of Giemsa staining is relatively straightforward (see page 113). Smears should be examined using an oil immersion objective. For the examination of cell cultures, a useful variation is to use dark ground illumination. Under these conditions the inclusions produce a yellow-green autofluorescence, allowing more rapid screening of slides. For clinical material, dark ground illumination is less useful owing to extraneous autofluorescence of other bacteria, or material such as alginate. By bright field microscopy, Giemsa stained inclusions give a blue ground-glass effect, the nuclei of the host cells staining purple.

Lugol's iodine staining is also simple to perform (*see* page 113). The specificity of the technique depends on the production of a glycogen matrix by the developing inclusion, which stains dark brown with iodine. Early inclusions may not have produced this matrix, and consequently may not stain. Stained inclusions appear as dark brown granular bodies against the pale cellular background. This method is of little use for the direct examination of genital material, owing to its intrinsic low sensitivity, and because extraneous dextrans in genital material will also take up the stain. The main use of this technique is for the rapid screening of cover slip cultures.

The use of indirect immunofluorescence of clinical material has, in some hands, proved nearly as reliable as cell culture, particularly in the diagnosis of endemic trachoma and infection of the male urethra. This is in contrast to other direct examination methods, which whilst adequate for the diagnosis of inclusion conjunctivitis (both adult and neonatal) are too insensitive for use in trachoma or genital infection. Immunofluorescence involves the preparation of specific antisera, the performance of the test, and the application of rigorous interpretative criteria, all of which are technically demanding and time consuming. The rapid fading of the stain prevents re-examination of slides at a later date. The principle of the method is to overlay the clinical material (fixed to a glass slide) with high titre, broadly reactive, hyperimmune serum. Following incubation and washing, the preparation is stained with a suitable fluorescein conjugated antiglobulin, and examined by fluorescence microscopy. Munday, *et al.* (1980) used indirect immunofluorescence following incubation of infected cycloheximide treated McCoy cells, and were able to produce culture results within twenty-four hours of inoculation of the cell line.

A description of the staining method, with technical details, is given in Schachter and Dawson (1978). Owing to the difficulties outlined above, this technique is for the present restricted to the major research centres.

Other staining techniques are primarily of research interest, or are still under development. A method analogous to the Giemsa technique is methylene blue staining which was described by Johnson, Chancerelle and Hobson (1978). Dark ground examination shows whitish blue inclusions. Machiavello's and Gimenez stains may be used for the examination of yolk sac material, or impression smears from clinical material, being of particular use for infections with *C. psittaci*. Acridine orange is a useful dye for studying the evolution of inclusions. During the formation of the initial bodies, the excess of RNA present causes the inclusions to stain red. With maturation of the inclusion, and the excess of DNA now present, the staining reaction is green. Recently Salari and Ward (1979) described a staining method using fluorescent DNA binding dyes. Inclusions are identifiable after eighteen hours of incubation in cell culture. However, the dyes used are expensive. Ashley, Richmond and Caul (1975) described the centrifugation of clinical material on to grids, followed by immunoferritin labelling, and the direct demonstration of inclusions by electron microscopy.

Isolation of *C. trachomatis*

For practical purposes, two methods of laboratory isolation are available. The earliest described technique is the use of fertilized hens' eggs yolk sac, as originally described by T'ang *et al.* (1957). This method has been superseded for routine isolations by cell culture techniques. The intracerebral, intranasal or intraperitoneal inoculation of mice whilst of use for *C. psittaci*, and occasionally as an animal model for *C. trachomatis* (Kuo and Chen, 1980), has no place in the routine isolation of *C. trachomatis*.

Yolk sac

The technique of isolating or propagating chlamydiae in the yolk sac of embryonated hens' eggs has become well established, but there are a number of drawbacks, not least of which is the problem of contamination. Both ocular and genital chlamydiae are frequently associated with other bacteria, both commensal and potentially pathogenic. The use of antimicrobial agents to protect cultures must be cautious; penicillin will prevent growth of the chlamydiae, whilst the aminoglycosides will not prevent superinfection of the eggs with, for example streptococci. The optimal isolation is obtained by the use of 7-day-old eggs obtained from an antibiotic-free source and incubated at 35°C. Even so, seasonal variation of susceptibility of hens' eggs is known to occur (Jawetz, 1962). Infected eggs are examined on the day of death, or the day prior to hatching, and the yolk sac smeared on a glass slide; this material is then stained and examined for elementary bodies. The sensitivity of the method is low, and serial blind passage is often required. This is time consuming, and may result in cross contamination of eggs (Harper, *et al.*, 1967; Dunlop, *et al.*, 1967). Yolk sac culture is still required for the production of high titre antigen for serological tests. The method, with technical details, is described by Schachter and Dawson (1978).

Cell culture

Because of the disadvantages of yolk sac culture, large scale isolation programmes were not possible until the development of cell culture techniques. Early experiments showed that egg-grown chlamydiae could be adapted to growth on suitable cell lines, for example HeLa cells (Furness, Graham and Reeve, 1960). However it was not until the work of Gordon and Quan in 1965 that the feasibility of cell culture for primary isolation of *C. trachomatis* from clinical specimens was demonstrated. A comparison of cell culture with yolk sac culture by Gordon, *et al.*, (1969) demonstrated the superiority of the cell culture, (41 per cent of clinical specimens yielded isolates with cell culture, compared to 8 per cent by yolk sac culture).

The two key stages in the processing of specimens for isolation in cell culture proved to be centrifugation of the inoculum on to the cell sheet and the use of host cells in a stationary non-dividing phase. Gordon and Quan used gamma irradiated McCoy cells; after irradiation, the cells were cultured on a glass microscope cover slip. This method produces a single cycle of growth for *C. trachomatis*, that is, on release of mature elementary bodies, further infection of host cells does not occur.

Centrifugation Centrifugation of the inoculum on to the cell culture enhances the entry of elementary bodies into the host cells. The centrifugation speeds recommended are probably insufficient physically to concentrate elementary bodies at the bottom of the tube. One possible explanation may be that elementary bodies close to the host cell sheet are normally repelled by the net negative charges on the cell and elementary body surfaces. This electrical force may be overcome by the centrifugal force applied.Diethyl-aminoethyl dextran (DEAE dextran), a polycation, similarly enhances the entry of elementary bodies into host cells (Rota and Nichols, 1971). The speed of centrifugation is not critical above about 3,000 G (Reeve, Owen and Oriel, 1975), although there is some evidence that low inoculum specimens may give a better yield when spun at 15,000 G (Darougar, Cubitt and Jones, 1974). The optimal temperature of centrifugation is between 35°C and 38°C, and care must be taken that the ambient temperature does not rise above 39°C.

Cell line and pre-treatment   The choice of cells has been the subject of much controversy. The mystique surrounding the McCoy cells is probably unfounded. Originally, these were derived from human synovial tissue to give a human fibroblastic cell line. However, at some unknown time the cells became indistinguishable both in karyotype and antigenicity from the mouse L929 tumour line, (Blyth and Taverne, 1974). Many cell lines have been employed, and a comparison of the sensitivity of eleven cell types was described by Croy, Kuo and Wang (1975), all cells being pre-treated with DEAE dextran. The cell lines currently in common use are McCoy, BHK (Baby Hamster Kidney) 21, and HeLa 229. Variation of sensitivity may be marked between batches of apparently identical cell lines, and it is important to acquire cells from laboratories which are actively isolating *C. trachomatis*.

The method of treatment of cells is largely a matter of personal preference. Moulder (1966) described how chlamydiae were energy parasites in the cell, and thus any agent which slows down metabolism in eukaryotic cells could be expected to favour the growth of prokaryotic chlamydiae. The method of Gordon and Quan used gamma irradiation, but any suitable source of radiation will suffice (e.g. gamma ray, beta ray, or electron beam). A disadvantage may be the difficulty of obtaining regular use of an irradiation source. This problem is obviated by the use of a cytotoxic agent, to render the cells either non-replicating, or not synthesizing macromolecules. Various methods have been reported, the first by Wentworth and Alexander (1974) using pretreatment of McCoy cells with 5-iodo-2-deoxy-uridine (IUDR). This method was later simplified by Reeve, Owen and Oriel (1975). IUDR is a thymine analogue, blocking DNA synthesis, and thus ultimately preventing cell division. At about the same time, Sompolinsky and Richmond (1974) described the use of cytochalasin B (a compound which inhibits cytoplasmic division) with McCoy cells. More recently, cycloheximide (an agent suppressing metabolism and reproduction in eukaryotic cells) has been used to treat McCoy cells (Ripa and Mårdh 1977). An advantage of this technique is that pretreatment of host cells before inoculation is not required; but in laboratories processing large numbers of specimens, this advantage is probably marginal. There would be obvious advantages if cells could be used without special treatment. Unirradiated, untreated BHK21 cells were compared favourably with irradiated McCoy cells by Blyth and Taverne (1974). Hobson, *et al.*, (1974) reported that irradiated, untreated McCoy cells were as sensitive as other cell culture systems. Other workers have been unable to confirm this, perhaps because inclusions in unirradiated, untreated cells are smaller, and require greater technical expertize to interpret, than in chemically treated cells.

Richmond (1976) suggested that host cell density was important, with the implication that if a high density of cells was used, a component for which *Chlamydia* and host cell compete might be selectively depleted by the host cell, to the detriment of the parasite. Conversely, non-replicating cells would not be synthesizing marcomolecules, allowing this essential component to be in excess, and available for the parasite. A low density of untreated host cells would be less likely to overwhelm the developing parasite. Hatch (1975) demonstrated that L-cell cultures of *C. psittaci* could be enhanced or inhibited by alteration in the concentration of isoleucine in the culture medium.

Untreated HeLa 229 cells augmented with DEAE dextran have been successfully used by Kuo, Wang *et al.* (1972), and this cell line was found to be the most sensitive of the eleven cell lines compared by Croy, Kuo and Wang (1975). Evans and Taylor-Robinson (1979) compared the advantages and disadvantages of the various cell treatments for a single batch of McCoy cells, which included cytochalasin B, IUDR, cycloheximide, emetine, hydrocortisone, irradiation and nontreatment. However, the differences between cycloheximide, cytochalasin B, and IUDR appear to be marginal.

The choice of culture method, and the staining procedure used (see page 113) is largely a matter of personal preference. The sensitivity between the accepted methods is similar, and once a method has been established in a laboratory, and is providing results comparable with other centres, it is wise to continue with it. All culture methods for *C. trachomatis* allow only a single cycle of growth to occur. To maintain cultures, it is necessary to passage on to fresh monolayers after about forty-eight hours. The routine use of passage for diagnosis is not warranted, as the increased yield does not justify the cost (Darougar *et al.*, 1972).

Counting inclusions is particularly labour intensive, and also unnecessary for routine purposes. The main use of inclusion counts is in the comparison of isolation techniques, using a single specimen to inoculate several different cell systems. Even here, other factors such as the size and character of inclusions, as well as the number of inclusions, must be taken into account. Details of the methods using IUDR and cycloheximide treated McCoy cells, are given on page 114.

Serological methods for the diagnosis of *C. trachomatis* infection

Culture techniques for *C. trachomatis* are expensive and labour intensive. The attractions of diagnosis by serological techniques are obvious. The clinician has always preferred a blood test for the diagnosis of infection rather than isolation attempts. Unfortunately, as is so often the case, the serological response to chlamydial infection is of only limited diagnostic use.

It is essential that when the usefulness of these serological tests for diagnosis is assessed at least one of the following criteria should be met:

1. Seroconversion, i.e. from no titre detectable in early tests to ≥8 later in the disease or during convalescence.
2. Greater than four-fold rise in antibody titre to IgG
3. Presence of IgM

In particular, a single estimation of antibody may only be of significance if the population studied is essentially seronegative.

Complement fixation test

The earliest method was a complement fixation test (CFT). Most methods in use are derived from the work of Meyer and Eddie (1964). They prepared a group antigen (*see* page 10), reacting to antibodies to both *C. trachomatis* and *C. psittaci*. Classically, *C. psittaci* antigen is used, prepared by boiling a phenolized culture. Schachter *et al.* (1967) compared CFT with non-serological methods in patients with oculo-genital infection, and found CFT to be the least useful diagnostic test. Whilst a regular rise in CF titre often occurred with acute genital infection in both men and women, patients were frequently seen late in the disease when titres were at a low level. This background level probably explained the difficulties encountered in the diagnosis of psittacosis. The same CF antigen was used in patients who may already have anti-chlamydial antibody from previous or current inapparent infection with *C. trachomatis*. In a further evaluation of diagnostic methods, Schachter *et al.* (1970) found that the CFT detected 44 per cent of ocular infections, but only 15 per cent of genital infections, when compared with direct Giemsa or fluorescent antibody staining of smears. Schachter and Dawson (1977) found that serum antibodies could be detected by micro-IF in 100 per cent of patients with inclusion conjunctivitis, but by CF in only 50 per cent of patients. The corresponding detection rates for chlamydial NGU were 90 per cent and 15 per cent, and for chlamydial cervicitis 99 per cent and 40 per cent. The CFT remains useful for the diagnosis of LGV and psittacosis, but is of no value for other oculo-genital infections with *C. trachomatis*.

Radio-immunoprecipitation test

A more sensitive radio-immunoprecipitation test (RIP) was developed by Gerloff and Watson (1967); it evolved from work being done on the detection of rickettsial antibodies. Like the CFT, the RIP is group specific, but approximately twenty times more sensitive (Philip, *et al.*, 1971). For this test a ^{32}P labelled meningopneumonitis (*C. psittaci*) antigen is used. In studies by Dwyer, *et al.* (1971), and Reeve, *et al.* (1974), the sensitivity of the RIP test was consistently better than the CFT, and comparable with the micro-IF test. Because of its serotype specificity, this latter has largely replaced the RIP, and is now the serological method of choice for studying chlamydial diseases.

Micro-immunofluorescence test

The micro-IF test was reported by Wang in 1971. Other workers had previously employed immunofluorescence, some achieving limited success in specificity (Bell and McComb, 1967). The micro-IF classically uses high titre egg yolk sac grown antigen, although cell grown antigen may also be used. Type specific antigens (*see* Table 2.2, page 11) are spotted on to a glass slide with the point of a pen nib. When dry, the antigen spots are overlaid with drops of suitably diluted patient's serum. Finally, a fluorescein labelled anti-human globulin (which may be of IgG, IgM or IgA specificity) is added, with the counterstain. The highest dilution of serum to demonstrate fluorescence expressed as a reciprocal is the titre of antibody present in the serum sample. Aetiological and epidemiological studies by this group (Wang and Grayston, 1974; Holmes, *et al.*, 1975) on patients with oculo-genital chlamydial infections, using the micro-IF test, demonstrated seroconversion to homologous strains, including the demonstration of type specific IgM antibody. However, the test is much too complicated to use for routine testing, hence much work has been carried out on simplification, and the use of pooled or cross-reacting antigens.

Wang, Grayston *et al.* (1975) divided the fifteen immunotypes into nine antigen pools, and used three dilutions of the patient's serum for screening purposes. Further reduction of the number of antigen pools was described by Treharne, Darougar and Jones (1977). Four antigen pools were used, arranged as follows:

1. Hyperendemic trachoma (serotypes A, B, C)
2. Paratrachoma/genital (serotypes D, E, F, G, H, I and K)
3. LGV (serotypes L1, L2 and L3)
4. Psittacosis

For routine use, the first three groups only are required. This method was found to be only slightly less sensitive than the classic micro-IF test, but with considerable saving in cost and technicians' time.

Treharne and his co-workers in common with many others noted that whilst the sensitivity of the micro-IF was high, the immunotype specificity was low. Cross reactions are frequent, and may complicate the determination of homologous antibody response in current infection. However, for routine diagnostic serological purposes, group specificity coupled with high sensitivity, are of greater importance than serotype specificity. These criteria are met by the RIP test, but the need for radio-immunoassay equipment limits the widespread use of the test. The cross reactions of serotypes are particularly noticeable with the LGV serotypes, and this fact has been exploited in the use of single antigens in the micro-IF test and its modifications, for example the use of the L2 serotype by Thomas, Reeve and Oriel, (1976).

Although cross reactions in the single antigen test are wide, their extent is variable. The single antigen test described by Thomas, Reeve and Oriel (1976) was negative in 4.5 per cent of sera which had been positive using an eleven serotype multiple antigen test. Richmond and Caul (1975) suggested that serotypes used in the single antigen tests probably detected a mixture of group and type specific antibody. The possible use of a cross-reacting antigen derived from reticulate body preparations was described by Yong *et al.* (1979). Reticulate bodies were separated out from host cells by the differential centrifugation of twenty-seven hour cultures. The preparations were found to be antigenically homologous, and when used as the antigen in a micro-IF test, demonstrated an excellent correlation between reticulate body antigen/antibody titre to a serotype C and elementary body antigen/antibody titres to all serotypes of *C. trachomatis*.

One of the major drawbacks to micro-IF is preparation of the antigen. Most methods use high titre egg-grown antigen. There are technical problems in preparing the antigen, even if the diagnostic laboratory has access to egg culture facilities. The use of cell grown antigen in the micro-IF test would therefore be one way of bringing micro-IF serotesting into the capabilities of a diagnostic laboratory. Richmond and Caul (1975) cultured *C. trachomatis* in wells on slides coated with polytetrafluorethylene. The cell grown mature inclusions thus produced were used as the antigen for an immunofluorescence test without further preparation, other than fixing the cells to the slides with acetone. Slides could then be stored in a moist environment until required. Test sera are added to the antigen-coated wells, and coupled to a suitable fluorescein conjugated antiglobulin. Single antigen screening tests, or type specific tests (including titration against the patient's own isolate), are obviously possible with this method (*see* page 115 for details).

Immunofluorescent techniques have been exploited to detect antibody in tears (Hanna, *et al.*, (1973); Darougar, *et al.*, 1978), and in genital tract secretions (Treharne, *et al.*, 1978). The significance of antibody detected in genital secretions will be discussed below.

The role of serology in the diagnosis of chlamydial infection

Serum antibody

The high prevalence of chlamydial antibody in sera was demonstrated by Wang, *et al.* (1975). An antibody titre ≥8 was detected in 60 per cent of adults (both male and female) attending an STD (sexually transmitted disease) clinic, in 25 per cent of adults with no history of genital infection and in 9 per cent of children under fifteen years of age. A survey of 360 patients attending an STD clinic, by Thomas, Reeve and Oriel (1976) detected antibody in one third, when a multiple antigen test was used. When a single cross-reacting antigen was used, 95 per cent of these positive sera demonstrated antibody. They concluded that a single antigen test was a useful screening test for chlamydial antibody.

Treharne, *et al.*, (1978) compared serology (both on serum and cervical secretions), with isolation, in an attempt to demonstrate that serology alone could be used to predict current chlamydial infection. A single specimen of serum or secretion was investigated. For serum, a titre of ≥64 for IgG (Treharne, Darougar and Jones 1977) and/or ≥8 for IgM was taken as diagnostic of current chlamydial infection. Isolates were obtained from 13 per cent of a group of unselected women attending an STD clinic, whilst 38 per cent had evidence of current chlamydial infection by serological results. These findings led the authors to conclude that serology was more sensitive than isolation. However, from their figures it would appear that had serology alone been used an appreciable number of the isolation positive women would have been excluded, as they did not have significant antibody levels in either serum or cervical secretion. Further studies by these workers (Simmons *et al.*, 1979; Treharne, *et al.*, 1979) attempted to predict current chlamydial infection in women with pelvic inflammatory disease. Unfortunately the results of

Chlamydia culture are not reported. These results must be interpreted with caution, as paired samples of serum or secretion were not examined.

A comparison of serum antibody with chlamydial isolation was described by Oriel *et al.* (1978), investigating women attending an STD clinic. Although an association between serum antibody and isolation of *C. trachomatis* from the cervix was demonstrated, over one third of the culture negative group had antibody ($\geqslant$16). A single cross reacting antigen was used in this study. Also using a single cross reacting antigen, Saikku and Paavonen (1978), found antibody significantly more often in isolation positive women, than in isolation negative groups; they noted that geometrical mean titres (which could reflect the ability of single estimations of antibody to differentiate these groups) did not differ significantly.

Demonstration of IgM antibodies might be a useful indicator of current chlamydial infection. However, because patients may present some time after infection, IgM may no longer be present in serum although *C. trachomatis* can be isolated from the patient. Alternatively, as Richmond andCaul (1975) have indicated, IgM may persist in some isolation negative patients. Further studies are clearly needed.

Local antibodies

The value of local antibodies as a diagnostic aid to chlamydial infection is controversial. Some workers have suggested that local antibody production is a good indicator of current chlamydial infection (Treharne, *et al.*, 1978). McComb *et al.* (1979) found serum antibody in 38 per cent of women college students, including 23 per cent of the sexually inexperienced. In contrast, cervical antibody was found only in the sexually experienced group, and correlated well with demonstrable infection of the cervix with *C. trachomatis*. It was concluded that local antibody was a better indicator for *C. trachomatis* infection than serum antibody. In contrast, Schachter, *et al.* (1979a) found that chlamydial antibodies whether detected by CF, or micro-IF, using serum or cervical secretions (IgG, IgM and IgA), were a poor indicator of current chlamydial infection when compared with cell culture. They thus concluded that serological diagnosis was unreliable. It is difficult to obtain cervical secretions that are not contaminated with blood. Further, evidence that local antibodies were locally produced, and not transudates from serum has been lacking. Richmond *et al.* (1980) examined serum and local antibodies from women attending an STD clinic. They noted a high correlation between the serum and local *Chlamydia* specific antibody, but a poor correlation between local antibody and the isolation of *Chlamydia* from the cervix. It was concluded that the cervical antibody was more probably derived from serum, than as a direct reponse to the cervical infection.

The discrepancies between the results outlined above indicate that at present the predictive value of single estimations of local or serum antibody for current chlamydial infection is doubtful, and isolation must remain the mainstay of diagnosis. However, the micro-IF test is a valuable aid to the understanding of chlamydial diseases, and some of the evidence for the pathogenicity of *C. trachomatis* is founded on results produced by this test. For the routine laboratory, where diagnosis not research is the requirement, there is little point in using the full micro-IF technique. At present, serology is only an aid to diagnosis (see page 109); it is more conveniently and economically performed using a single antigen test, either in the micro-IF, or the whole inclusion test of Richmond and Caul (1975). Serial estimations are required to demonstrate a diagnostic change in titre. Single estimations are notoriously unreliable, not only in chlamydial infections, but in all infections where serological diagnosis must be used. Idealy, an IF test should be used to back titrate the patient's sera (or local secretions) against the patient's own isolate. Evidence of a rise in titre to a homologous strain is unequivocal.

Other serological techniques

Newer techniques of antibody detection have been investigated by several workers. Countercurrent immuno-electrophoresis (CIE) was investigated as a diagnostic test for LGV by Caldwell and Kuo (1977). They found that 95 per cent of patients with clinical evidence of LGV had antibody, but could not detect antibody by CIE in fifty patients with NGU, although thirty-eight of these had demonstrable antibody by micro-IF. Thus it would appear that this test is not sensitive enough for the diagnosis of chlamydial NGU. Enzyme-linked immunosorbent assay (ELISA) was used by Lewis, Thacker and Mitchell (1977). Only patients with psittacosis or LGV were investigated, and they found that patients seropositive by CF had a high titre by ELISA. Other tests are available, for example single radial haemolysis, but the assessments of their usefulness have yet to be published.

Comment

The various laboratory methods for diagnosing oculo-genital infection with *C. trachomatis* are summarized in Table 3.1, along with an indication of their usefulness. Cell culture remains the most reliable and convenient technique for the routine laboratory. It is important that cell lines are obtained from a source actively isolating chlamydiae, and that reagents are checked to ensure they are not inhibitory to the cells or the parasite. Direct examination of clinical material is often of use in neonatal conjunctivitis, particularly when laboratory facilities are not readily available. In this situation, iodine or Giemsa staining is most convenient.

The role of serology in diagnosis is considerably less certain. The status of local antibodies is, to say the least, equivocal. The background prevalence of serum antibody in the general population is high, hence antibody determination may not reflect current infection. Patients may present late in the disease, and thus not show IgM or seroconversion. We have little knowledge of the time course for the development of anti-chlamydial antibody. It is difficult to ensure that patients return for follow-up studies, reducing the chances of demonstrating change in the serological titre. Infections are often recurrent, and it may be impossible to determine whether this is due to relapse or re-infection.

Serological screens of various populations have added much to our know-

Table 3.1 Laboratory diagnosis of oculo-genital chlamydial infection

	Cytology			Culture		Serology (CFT)	Serology (micro-IF)		
	Giemsa	Iodine	IF	Yolk sac	Cell		Serum IgG (single estimate)	Serum IgM	Local Ab
NGU	+/-	-	+	+/-	++	-	+/-	+	?
Cervicitis	+/-	-	+	+/-	++	-	+/-	+	+/-
Infant inclusion conjunctivitis	++	+	++	++	++	-	+	++	+
Adult inclusion conjunctivitis	+	+/-	++	+	++	-	+	+	+
Pneumonitis	+/-	+/-	+/-	+/-	++	-	++	++	?
LGV	-	-	-	++	++	+	+	?	?

++, Useful; +, Occasionally useful; +/-, Unlikely to be useful; -, Useless; ?, Not known ledge of chlamydial infection, but are of little use for predicting active infection with *C. trachomatis*. It is easy to expect too much from a serological test, on what is usually a superficial infection. Systemic diseases, such as LGV, pneumonitis, and endocarditis would be expected to produce the best serological response, and this is demonstrated well with LGV. Indeed, in all three diseases noted, serology may be the only means of diagnosis available. For the common oculo-genital syndromes, serology has a long way to go before it can be said to aid the routine diagnosis of *C. trachomatis* infection.

4

Eye infections

There are two major forms of chlamydial eye disease. **Trachoma (blinding trachoma, hyperendemic trachoma)** has its greatest prevalence in North Africa, the Middle East and the Far East. It is a chronic inflammatory eye disease which may lead to conjunctival and corneal scarring, and it is the commonest cause of preventable blindness in the world. **Paratrachoma** comprises adult inclusion conjunctivitis, diffuse punctate keratitis and **endemic** trachoma. It is common in Western urban societies, and it is associated with genital infection through direct or indirect contact with genital material. Neonatal inclusion conjunctivitis is also due to infection by genital strains of *C. trachomatis*, acquired from the mother during birth.

Trachoma

In hyperendemic areas trachoma is caused by serotypes A, B, Ba and C of *C. trachomatis*. Transmission is from eye to eye, often via vectors such as flies, and the disease is always worse in poor countries. Trachoma begins in childhood, and young children contribute most to the reservoir of chlamydial infection in trachomatous areas. This reservoir favours frequent reinfection of the eye by *C. trachomatis* through 'ocular promiscuity' (Jones, 1975).

The clinical features of trachoma are usually described as occurring in four stages, but Jones (1964) depicts a preliminary stage of acute or subacute conjunctivitis with diffuse hyperaemia, oedema and conjunctival infiltration. This progresses to trachoma Stage 1 with the appearance of lymphoid follicles; although initially these appear on both the lower and upper tarsal conjunctivae they later become more prominent inside the upper lid. Papillary hyperplasia develops in the conjunctival epithelium, and punctate keratitis with a diffuse infiltration and formation of new blood vessels in the cornea (pannus) occurs. The disease now passes to the chronic stage, trachoma Stage 2. Follicles are now readily visible, and corneal infiltration and pannus increase to a maximum. The appearance of small stellate scars on the conjunctiva heralds the appearance of trachoma Stage 3. Cicatrization now occurs to a variable extent, and if involvement of the upper lid is severe may lead to entropion and corneal ulceration. After some years the inflammatory process resolves to leave a permanently damaged eye — Stage 4 trachoma. Resolution of the follicles leaves small limbal depressions (Herbert's pits).

The course of trachoma is greatly influenced by the presence of other bacterial infections as well as by late re-infection by *C. trachomatis*. In particular, *Haemophilus aegyptius* (Koch-Weeks bacillus), *Moraxella lacunata* (Morax-Axenfeld diplobacillus), gonococcal and staphylococcal infections facilitate the onset of trachoma, aggravate its course, and delay or prevent healing (Majčuk, 1976). The association of other bacteria with *C. trachomatis* to produce severe disease is of particular interest in view of recent work on experimental chlamydial infection in the cat (Darouger *et al.*, 1978, and *see* page 20).

Inclusion conjunctivitis and related diseases

Inclusion conjunctivitis and its related syndromes are usually due to infection by genital strains of *C. trachomatis*, usually serotypes D to K. Occasionally ocular strains, serotypes B, Ba and C, which cross-react with genital strains, are recovered. Infection of the eye occurs by direct contact with genital material during orogenital sexual relations, or through the transfer of such material by the hands or by other means. *C. trachomatis* has been isolated from the cervix in up to 90 per cent of women and from the urethra in 50 per cent of men with paratrachoma (Darougar *et al.*, 1972). Thus the prevalence of ocular infection with genital chlamydiae is linked to sexual promiscuity. Accidental infection has, however, been described, eg of gynaecologists whose eyes have been splashed with genital exudate during surgery. It is interesting that inclusion conjunctivitis is said to be very rare among male homosexuals (Schachter and Dawson, 1978), since some workers have reported that chlamydial infection of the urethra is likewise uncommon in this group (see page 43). Inclusion conjunctivitis was at one time called 'swimming bath conjunctivitis' (Fehr, 1900), but the identification of this syndrome with *C. trachomatis* is not certain; some infections may have been with adenoviruses, which are also associated with swimming baths.

The incubation period of adult inclusion conjunctivitis is one to two weeks. In most cases only one eye is affected. The onset is with discomfort, lacrimation and conjunctival erythema. After about two weeks the disease is at its worst, and mucopurulent discharge, marked hyperaemia and multiple lymphoid follicles are all present. In contrast to trachoma, the follicles are mostly on the lower lid. At this stage pre-auricular lymphadenopathy may be seen and some patients show signs of upper respiratory tract infection. Corneal involvement is common in inclusion conjunctivitis; diffuse punctate keratitis occurs in many patients, and subepithelial infiltrates may last for several months.

Adult oculo-genital chlamydial infections run a fluctuating but ultimately self-limiting course. However, residual conjunctival scarring is not unusual, and some cases progresses to a clinical picture indistinguishable from trachoma, with pannus and characteristic scar formation. The development of trachomatous features in some cases of adult inclusion conjunctivitis is analogous to the appearance of pannus, conjunctival follicles and scarring as a late complication of neonatal inclusion conjunctivitis (Grayston and Wang, 1975). The family resemblance between some of the clinical features of adult and neonatal inclusion conjunctivitis on the one hand and trachoma on the other should not obscure the fact that epidemiology and natural history of trachoma and paratrachoma are really quite different.

Neonatal inclusion conjunctivitis broadly resembles the adult disease, and is due to infection by the same serotypes of *C. trachomatis*. Some infants yielding chlamydiae from the conjunctival sac show no clinical evidence of infection, but in most cases a clinically apparent disease is present. This varies greatly in severity; in some infected babies there is only a mild conjunctivitis, a 'sticky eye', but in others there is a severe purulent ophthalmia (Figs. 4.1 and 4.2). The physical signs of neonatal inclusion conjunctivitis include conjunctival erythema, a watery discharge which may become purulent, particularly if secondary infection occurs, and oedema of the eyelids. In some cases 'pseudomembranes', which are due to inflammatory exudate adherent to the conjunctiva, are present. Lymphoid follicles are a later development, and usually appear after the age of 3 weeks (Freedman *et al.*, 1966).

It was formerly believed that neonatal inclusion conjunctivitis was a mild disease which resolved in a few weeks or months without sequelae, but although this is the usual outcome it is not invariable. Conjunctival scarring and superficial corneal vascularization were seen in 10 of 38 cases studied in Moorfields Eye Hospital in London by Freedman *et al.* in 1966. No lid deformities have been seen, but pannus can sometimes occur. These signs may persist for months or even years so that eventually a trachoma-like disease ensues (Watson and Gairdner, 1968). Conversely, some eye conditions in older children which clinically appear to be non-endemic trachoma may yield conjunctival isolates of genital D-E serotypes of *C. trachomatis*; it is possible that these cases are due to a continuing infection which began in the neonatal period (Grayston and Wang, 1975).

In trachoma, secondary infection by other organisms greatly influences the clinical disease, and the same may be true of neonatal inclusion conjunctivitis. *Staph. aureus*, *Klebsiella*, *Pseudomonas* and other Gram-negative

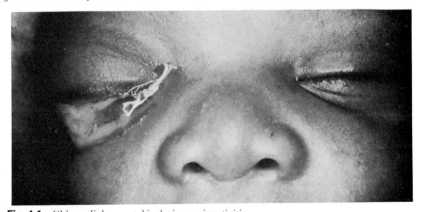

Fig. 4.1 Chlamydial neonatal inclusion conjunctivitis

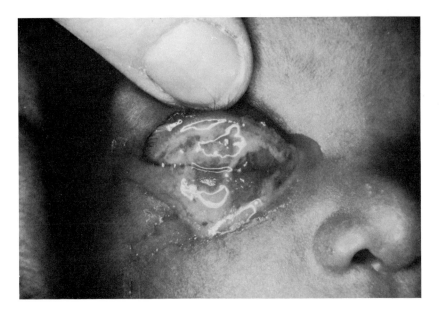

Fig. 4.2   Conjunctival hyperaemia and oedema in neonatal inclusion conjunctivitis

bacteria are usually nosocomial, but streptococci, *Haemophilus* spp. and other nasopharyngeal organisms are more often derived from family members. The effects of these organisms are hard to assess, since they may be found in normal eyes. Nevertheless, most physicians believe that secondary infection aggravates inclusion conjunctivitis in neonates, and it may in addition promote an earlier age of onset (Rees *et al.*, 1977c). It must not be forgotten that *C. trachomatis* and *N. gonorrhoeae* may co-exist in some cases of ophthalmia neonatorum, as indeed they do in both the male and female genital tract.

5

Genital infections of man

By far the commonest chlamydial infection of the genital tract in men is NGU; PGU is closely related and is also common. In young men, epididymitis may often be caused by *C. trachomatis*. As yet there is no evidence that chlamydiae are involved in the pathogenesis of prostatitis but chlamydial proctitis occurs in homosexual men. These diseases will now be considered in turn.

Non-gonococcal urethritis

In England, over 70 000 cases of NGU are diagnosed each year in STD clinics. The number of cases reported has been steadily increasing for many years (Fig. 5.1) and is twice as common as gonococcal urethritis. Typically, a man with NGU presents with a history of urethral irritation and dysuria, followed by the appearance of a mucoid or mucopurulent urethral discharge. The symptoms begin one to two weeks after intercourse, usually with a new partner. The diagnosis is made by demonstrating significant leucocytosis on a Gram-stained urethral smear or in a first-catch specimen of urine, and excluding *N. gonorrhoeae* by microscopy and culture. When patients have obvious symptoms and signs the diagnosis is easy, but patients with mild infections give more difficulty. In order to avoid over-diagnosis, a lower level for significant leucocytosis must be defined, and many physicians now accept 4–5 polymorphonuclear leucocytes (PMN) per high-power field ($\times$ 100 objective) as significant (Swartz *et al.*, 1978). Previous definitions in terms of >20 PMN per field are certainly too restrictive. It is preferable to collect specimens not less than two hours after urination to obtain reasonable uniformity of conditions, particularly for follow-up after treatment. The enumeration of PMN in first-catch urine after centrifugation and resuspension is used by some workers. Thus Holmes *et al.* (1975) centrifuged the first 10 ml of voided urine and resuspended the deposit in 0.5 ml urine. One drop of this was then examined at magnification $\times$ 400, $\geqslant$20 PMN per field being taken as diagnostic of significant pyuria. Whether this method, examination of a Gram-stained smear, or both are used is a matter of personal choice. Some physicians restrict the diagnosis of NGU to patients who have a visible urethral discharge, but since mild and symptomless infections are quite common, too rigid a definition in terms of one physical sign will exclude some infected patients. Indeed, in some men a significant leucocytosis is apparent only after the patient has refrained from urination overnight (Rodin, 1971), and *C. trachomatis* has been recovered from the urethra of some men in these circumstances.

Epidemiologically, NGU behaves as a sexually transmitted disease, but its aetiology has always been doubtful and even now is not completely understood, several infecting micro-organisms and probably some host factors being involved (Table 5.1). Today, *C. trachomatis* is considered to be the most important cause of NGU, but this organism cannot account for more than 50–60 per cent of cases. *T. vaginalis* and Herpes simplex virus can undoubtedly cause NGU, but in Western Europe and North America these organisms are responsible for less than 5 per cent of infections. It is likely that there are other infecting organisms, and that these are sensitive to tetracyclines; whether *Ureaplasma urealyticum*, or other organisms not identified, are involved in the aetiology of NGU remains to be seen.

Isolation of *C. trachomatis* from men with NGU

Examination of urethral specimens from men with NGU was one of the first investigations attempted when cell culture techniques for *C. trachomatis*

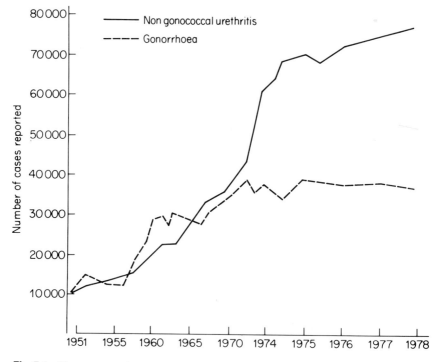

Fig. 5.1   Non-gonococcal urethritis and gonorrhoea reported cases (England and Wales) 1951–1978

Table 5.1 Aetiology of nongonococcal urethritis

Organism	Percentage of cases caused
Chlamydia trachomatis	35–60
Ureaplasma urealyticum ⎫ Other bacteria ⎭	uncertain
Trichomonas vaginalis ⎫ Herpes simplex virus ⎭	<5

became available, and many studies from Europe and North America have now appeared (Table 5.2). The isolation rates vary between 30 and 58 per cent. In other areas, data on its incidence in urethral infection is scanty, but it may be lower in the Far East (Gale *et al.*, 1970).

There are several variables which affect the isolation rate for *C. trachomatis* within a group of men with NGU:

1. *The composition of the group.* Some studies have shown a much lower incidence of *Chlamydia*-positive NGU in homosexual men than in heterosexuals. Bowie, Alexander and Holmes (1978) recovered *C. trachomatis* from only 2 (13 per cent) of 15 men with homosexually acquired NGU, and Goldmeier and Darougar (1977) refer to the isolation of chlamydiae from only 2 (5 per cent) of 39 similar men. The evidence is conflicting, since another group of workers recovered *C. trachomatis* from 7 (32 per cent) of 22 homosexual men with NGU (Oriel, *et al.*, 1976).

2. *Recent administration of antimicrobial agents.* It is obviously necessary in these prevalence studies not to include men who have recently taken antimicrobial agents (the usual limit is one month before examination), as these may significantly affect the isolation rate.

3. *Duration of urethritis.* Both Richmond, Hilton and Clarke (1972) and Oriel, Reeve *et al.* (1976) have reported higher isolation in men with NGU who had symptoms for seven days or more than in men whose symptoms were of less than seven days duration.

4. *The technique of specimen collection.* Endourethral swabs or curettes yield more positive results than meatal swabs, and doctors obtain more rewarding specimens than nursing staff (Dunlop, Vaughan-Jackson and Darougar, 1972).

5. *The time between specimen collection and inoculation of the cell monolayer.* This should be as short as possible. After storage at +4°C for twenty-four hours the isolation rate declines sharply; storage at −70°C may also give a lower isolation rate (Reeve, Owen and Oriel, 1975).

6. *The sensitivity of the isolation procedure.* This is affected by the cell line used, the method of pre-treatment of the cells, the speed of centrifugation of clinical specimens on to the monolayers, and the temperature of centrifugation (see page 27).

7. *Repeated specimen collection.* Evidence on this point is conflicting. Perroud and Miedzybrodzka (1978) report that they raised their isolation rate by 9 per cent through taking one extra specimen, but Holmes *et al.* (1975) obtained no additional positive results through repeated specimen collection. Even in those cases where additional isolates are obtained it is not clear whether this is because of repeated examinations *per se* or because a lapse of time allows a

Table 5.2 Results of cell culture for C. trachomatis in men with non-gonococcal urethritis and men without urethritis

Country	Authors	Men with NGU		Control men	
		Number yielding chlamydia/number tested	Percentage positive	Number yielding chlamydia/number tested	Percentage positive
UK	Dunlop, Vaughan-Jackson et al. (1972b)	44/99	44		
UK	Oriel et al., (1972)	49/135	36	0/31	0
UK	Richmond, Hilton and Clarke, (1972)	40/103	39	5/92	5
UK	Oriel et al., (1976)	118/240	49	3/60	5
UK	Prentice, Taylor-Robinson and Csonka, (1976)	43/136	32		
UK	Alani et al., (1977)	116/385	30		
UK	Coufalik, Taylor-Robinson and Csonka, (1979)	93/217	43		
USA	Schachter et al., (1975a)	24/42	57	0/57	0
USA	Holmes et al., (1975)	48/113	42	4/58	7
USA	Wong et al., (1977)	21/67	31	3/85	4
USA	Bowie et al., (1977)	23/69	33	1/39	3
USA	Swartz et al., (1978)	35/107	33	6/112	5
Sweden	Johannisson, Sernyd and Lycke, (1977)	162/367	43		
Switzerland	Perroud and Miedzybrodzka (1978)	124/238	52	1/40	3
Finland	Paavonen et al., (1978a)	39/75	52		
Finland	Terho (1978a)	93/159	58	0/64	0

higher concentration of organisms within the urethra. Urethral isolates of *C. trachomatis* from men with NGU have been immunotyped by several investigators (Table 5.3). Serotypes D-E and F-G are the commonest.

Table 5.3 Results of immunotyping urethral isolates of *C. trachomatis* from men with non-gonococcal urethritis

Author	Number of isolates	Number of immunotypes						
		B	D-E	F-G	C-J	H	I	K
Holmes *et al.,* (1975)	50	2	22	16	3	3	2	2
Bowie *et al.,* (1977)	22	0	16	4	1	0	1	0
Perroud and Miedzybrodzka, (1978)	35	0	18	10	1	0	0	6

Isolation of *C. trachomatis* from men without urethritis

For valid comparisons to be made on chlamydial isolation rates, it is important that the composition of control groups of men without urethritis is carefully defined. First, they should match the NGU groups in age, ethnic origin, sexual orientation (there should not be a higher proportion of homosexuals in either group), and sexual activity as indicated by the number of partners within an arbitrary time of six to twelve months. Second, urethritis should be excluded by examination two hours after micturition, or in the morning after the patient has held urine overnight; this precaution is particularly necessary because of the frequent occurrence of mild infections.

These requirements have not always been fully met in the published studies, but it is clear that men without urethritis show a very low level of chlamydial infection in comparison with men with NGU (*see* Table 5.2).

Antibodies against *C. trachomatis* in men with NGU

The majority of men with *Chlamydia*-positive NGU have serum antibodies demonstrable by immunofluorescence. Positive results (titres ≥8) have been reported in 70–100 per cent of these patients; in contrast, the proportion of seroreactors among men with *Chlamydia*-negative NGU is lower, 18–44 per cent (Reeve *et al.*, 1974; Holmes *et al.*, 1975; Bowie, Alexander and Holmes, 1977; Richmond and Caul, 1977). These data must be interpreted with the knowledge that chlamydial antibodies are present in over 50 per cent of unselected men attending some STD clinics (Reeve *et al.*, 1974; Grayston and Wang, 1975).

Evidence of recent microbial infection is normally provided not by a single determination of IgG antibody titre but by the presence of IgM antibody, a rising titre of IgG antibody, or by seroconversion. IgM antibodies have been found in 28–30 per cent of men with *Chlamydia*-positive NGU and in 3–8 per cent of men with *Chlamydia*-negative NGU (Reeve *et al.*, 1974; Holmes *et al.*, 1975; Richmond and Caul, 1977). Rising titres and seroconversion have been difficult to demonstrate in men with NGU because of high background levels of antibody and the practical problems of collecting serial specimens from patients in STD clinics. Holmes *et al.* (1975) demonstrated a fourfold rise in titre in 11 (31 per cent) of 36 men with *Chlamydia*-positive NGU but in only 2 (4 per cent) of 50 men with *Chlamydia*-negative NGU. Seroconversion (titre $<8\rightarrow>16$) was noted in 7 (54 per cent) of 13 *Chlamydia*-positive and in one (4 per cent) of 25 *Chlamydia*-negative patients.

The most convincing serological evidence of chlamydial infection in NGU has come from studies of men who are experiencing their first attack of urethritis. Bowie, Alexander and Holmes (1977) found seroconversion in 9 of 10 such men with *Chlamydia*-positive NGU who had had symptoms for up to ten days, but in only 1 of 10 who had had symptoms for longer. Seroconversion was observed in only 1 of 13 men with *Chlamydia*-negative NGU. IgM antibodies were detected in 16 of 20 men with *Chlamydia*-positive NGU and in 3 of 39 with *Chlamydia*-negative NGU. Paavonen *et al.* (1978a), using a single-antigen immuno-fluorescence method, reported a fourfold or greater rise in titre in 8 of 17 men with *Chlamydia*-positive NGU but in none of 7 who were *Chlamydia*-negative.

Although serology seems to have limited value in the diagnosis of chlamydial urethral infection except in special circumstances, there is no doubt that antibody responses do occur in men with *Chlamydia*-positive NGU. These responses in themselves are not, of course, proof of pathogencity.

Selective therapy of NGU

It has never been proposed that *C. trachomatis* is the only cause of NGU, and other infective agents must be concerned. Of these, *Ureaplasma urealyticum* has attracted the most interest; while not having the importance of *C. trachomatis* it may well cause some infections. When the roles of this organism and of *C. trachomatis* in NGU were being studied it was realized that the differences in their response to antibacterial agents could be exploited to provide evidence for the bacterial pathogenesis of NGU. Selective eradication of *C. trachomatis* appears to correlate with clinical improvement. Bowie *et al.* (1976) treated a group of men with NGU with either sulphafurazole (which is active against *C. trachomatis* but inactive against *U. urealyticum*) or with spectinomycin (which has no action against *C. trachomatis* although it is active against *U. urealyticum*). Seven men with *Chlamydia*-positive NGU were treated with sulphafurazole, the organism was eradicated in all of them, and all showed clinical improvement. Conversely, when 4 men with *Chlamydia*-positive NGU were treated with spectinomycin, chlamydiae were re-isolated in all of them, and none showed clinical improvement. In a placebo-controlled study, Prentice, Taylor-Robinson and Csonka (1976) found that patients with *Chlamydia*-associated NGU responded significantly better to minocycline than to a placebo. Finally, Coufalik, Taylor-Robinson and Csonka (1979) conducted similar experiments using either minocycline (which is active against *C. trachomatis* and *U. urealyticum*) or rifampicin (which is active only against *C. trachomatis*). In general the responses to therapy in all these studies were as would be expected if both *C. trachomatis* and *U. urealyticum* cause NGU, although an aetiological role for either organism cannot be proved by these means.

Comment

It is now accepted that there is compelling evidence that *C. trachomatis* is an important cause of NGU. This evidence has come from several sources: the isolation of chlamydiae from men with NGU in comparison with control groups, serology of *Chlamydia*-associated NGU and studies of the effects of treatment have been reviewed above. Further evidence comes from the markedly greater prevalence of chlamydial infection of the cervix in female contacts of men with *Chlamydia*-positive NGU than in contacts of men with *Chlamydia*-negative NGU (see page 53). Finally, some animal experiments have shown that genital strains of *C. trachomatis* induce urethritis in some primates (Digiacomo *et al.*, 1975). Thus although no human inoculations have been performed Koch's postulates may be regarded as having been satisfied, all the available evidence points in the same direction, and there can no longer be any doubt that *C. trachomatis* can cause urethritis. This urethritis may, of course, be primary or secondary. The latter is exemplified by PGU (*see* below). It is assumed that in NGU *C. trachomatis* is behaving as a primary invader; it could only be regarded as a secondary infecting organism in those cases where a primary pathogen could be identified. Since no evidence of this kind has come to light, we regard this matter as speculative, and see no reason to question the generally held view that in men with *Chlamydia*-positive NGU *C. trachomatis* is the primary cause of the urethritis and should be treated as such.

Clinical signs of NGU

The symptoms and signs of urethritis vary with the inflammatory response to infective challenge. Although this is not invariable, gonorrhoea has a shorter incubation period than NGU, and the discharge is more often profuse and purulent; a clinical diagnosis of gonococcal urethritis is often possible. Differences between chlamydial and non-chlamydial NGU might be anticipated, but unfortunately the evidence is contradictory and unhelpful.

There is no difference between the incubation period of *Chlamydia*-positive and *Chlamydia*-negative NGU (Oriel *et al.*, 1972; Tehro, 1978a). Some investigators have seen an association between the presence of chlamydiae and severe urethritis, shown by a profuse purulent discharge (Richmond, Hilton and Clarke, 1972; Schachter *et al.*, 1975a; Alani *et al.*, 1977; Terho, 1978a). Others find the reverse, chlamydial infection being associated with mild urethritis (Holmes, *et al.*, 1975; Bowie *et al.*, 1977). Many physicians can find no differences between men with *Chlamydia*-positive and *Chlamydia*-negative NGU (Oriel, Reeve *et al.*, 1976; Perroud and Miedzybrodzka, 1978).

A physical sign of possible diagnostic significance was described by Dunlop *et al.* (1967, 1971a), who found follicles in the mucous membrane of the terminal urethra with the aid of an operating microscope; these were of similar appearance to the follicles seen in patients with inclusion conjunctivitis. This interesting observation has not been pursued further in controlled studies, so it is not possible to say whether or not these follicles are a reliable diagnostic aid.

Post-gonococcal urethritis

The definition of PGU is persistent or recurrent urethritis, not caused by *N. gonorrhoeae*, occurring in men after the treatment of gonorrhoea. The precise diagnostic criteria used are variable. Some workers diagnose PGU one week after the treatment of gonorrhoea but others wait for two weeks; some require a visible urethral discharge for diagnosis, others do not; and there are variations, as with NGU, in the level of urethral leucocytosis which is regarded as significant. A reasonable definition of PGU is the presence, two weeks after treatment of gonorrhoea, of at least 4–5 PMN per high power field in specimens collected ⩾ two hours after urination, and/or equivalent pyuria, regardless of whether a urethral discharge can be seen. Culture for *N. gonorrhoeae* is, by definition, negative. Thus the diagnostic criteria for PGU and NGU are similar, and indeed PGU is generally regarded as the result of a mixed infection with *N. gonorrhoeae* and one or more of the agents which cause NGU; these agents are for the most part unresponsive to the single dose treatment with penicillin derivatives or spectinomycin which is generally used for gonorrhoea. If penicillin is used for treating gonorrhoea, PGU is quite common and will develop in between one-quarter and one-third of cases.

Richmond, Hilton and Clarke (1972) were the first to demonstrate an association between PGU and *C. trachomatis* in a large series. This association has now been amply confirmed (Table 5.4). The isolation rate of *C. trachomatis* from the urethra in gonococcal urethritis varies between 11–32 per cent. This rather wide range may be due in part to differences in the composition of the study groups, particularly in the proportion of homosexuals. As with NGU, there seems to be a lower prevalence of *C. trachomatis* in men with homosexually acquired gonorrhoea than in those with heterosexually acquired infections; this difference is particularly marked in the USA (Bowie, Alexander and Holmes, 1978).

It has been observed that some men with gonorrhoea yield chlamydiae from the urethra after, although not before, antibiotic therapy. The increase in the isolation rate may be due simply to the advantage of repeating a biological test, but it is more probable that the passage of time between the first and second attempts allows a higher concentration of chlamydial organisms to develop (see page 9). Whatever the explanation, the effects are shown in Table 5.5.

Serology of *Chlamydia*-associated PGU

Serology has not been very helpful in establishing that *C. trachomatis* can cause PGU. IgG antibody was found in 15 (100 per cent) of 15 men with *Chlamydia*-positive PGU and in 2 (25 per cent) of 11 with *Chlamydia*-negative PGU by Oriel *et al.* (1975b). Vaughan-Jackson *et al.* (1977) found IgG antibody in 11 (48 per cent) of 23 men with *Chlamydia*-positive PGU and in 6 (29 per cent) of 21 men with *Chlamydia*-negative PGU; IgM antibody was found in 8 (73 per cent) of 11 men with IgG antibody and positive cultures and in 1 (16 per cent) of 6 of the men with negative cultures. Attempts to demonstrate rises in titre were unsuccessful.

Table 5.4 Isolation of C. trachomatis from men with gonococcal urethritis before and after antibiotic therapy

| Country | Authors | Pre-treatment | | Treatment | Post-treatment | | | |
| | | Number yielding chlamydiae/ number tested | Percentage positive | | With PGU | | Without PGU | |
					Number yielding chlamydiae/ number tested	Percentage positive	Number yielding chlamydiae/ number tested	Percentage positive
UK	Richmond, Hilton and Clarke (1972)	32/99	32	Penicillin Gentamicin Kanamycin	17/21	81	10/46	22
UK	Oriel et al., (1975b)	11/44	25	Gentamicin	15/26	58	0/18	0
UK	Oriel, et al., (1976)	12/46	26	Ampicillin	15/17	88	3/29	10
UK	Oriel et al., (1977)	11/63	17.5	Spectinomycin	17/25	68	0/38	0
UK	Vaughan-Jackson et al., (1977)	20/95	21	Penicillin Kanamycin	26/49	53	0/17	0
USA	Holmes et al., (1975)	13/69	19	Penicillin Ampicillin Spectinomycin	11/20	55	0/13	0
USA	Bowie et al., (1978)	23/121	19	Penicillin Ampicillin Amoxycillin	10/26	38	0/20	0
Switzerland	Perroud and Miedzybrodzka (1978)	32/139	23	Thiamphenicol	15/19	79	5/10	50

Comment

The majority of infections with gonorrhoea are treated with single-dose therapy: benzyl or procaine penicillin with or without probenecid, ampicillin with probenecid, or spectinomycin are the agents most commonly used. All these regimens have little effect on *C. trachomatis*, which can be re-isolated (or isolated for the first time) after therapy in the majority of cases, almost invariably in association with PGU (*see* Table 5.4). When usual treatment schedules are used, *C. trachomatis* is responsible for between one half and two thirds of PGU. The failure of commonly used therapy for gonorrhoea to eliminate *C. trachomatis* from the genital tract has important implications for both men and women, which will be discussed later (see page 95).

Table 5.5   Isolation of *C. trachomatis* from men with gonococcal urethritis: effect of repeated specimen collection

	Percentage isolation rate	
Author	First attempt	All attempts
Holmes *et al.*, (1975)	19	33
Oriel *et al.*, (1976)	26	33
Terho, (1978b)	29	42

Epididymitis

In older men epididymitis is associated with urinary tract infections, and is usually seen as a complication of urinary obstruction or after prostatic surgery. In younger men, however, these causes are not operative; some cases are caused by *N. gonorrhoeae* and a few by *M. tuberculosis*, but the aetiology of the remainder has been doubtful.

The first suggestion that *C. trachomatis* might be a cause of epididymitis was made by Heap (1975), who noted a significant rise in titre of group-reactive antibodies to *Chlamydia* in two men with acute epididymitis. Harnisch *et al.* (1977) performed detailed microbiology on twenty-four men with acute epididymitis. Six were aged 45 years or more; four of these men had urinary tract infections with *Esch. coli*, *Klebsiella* or *Ps. aeruginosa*, but no urethral isolates of *N. gonorrhoeae* or *C. trachomatis* were made. Eighteen men were aged 32 years or less; six men yielded isolates of *N. gonorrhoeae* from the urethra and six *C. trachomatis*, while one man yielded both organisms; no enterobacteria were recovered. Three paired sera were available from the men with chlamydial infections, two of which showed a fourfold rise in micro-IF titre.

This work showed that urethral infection by *C. trachomatis* could be associated with epididymitis, and indicated the possibility that the organism might cause the disease. More direct aetiological studies were performed by Berger *et al.* (1978), who investigated sixteen men with epididymitis, from all of whom they obtained epididymal aspirates. Ten men were aged 35 years or more; no epididymal isolates of *N. gonorrhoeae* or *C. trachomatis* were obtained, but coliforms (*Esch. coli* with or without *Proteus mirabilis*) were recovered from 5 of the 10 men. Six men were aged less than 35 years. Epididymal aspirates yielded chlamydiae in 5 of them, but all were negative for *N. gonorrhoeae*; no urinary coliforms were found. This study also showed that the majority of men with *Chlamydia*-associated epididymitis also showed evidence of NGU, but the absence of urethritis and failure to culture *C. trachomatis* from the urethra did not exclude chlamydial infection of the epididymis.

Comment

These studies confirm that the pathogenesis of epididymitis in older men is linked with urinary tract infection. In younger men, the recovery of *C. trachomatis* not only from the urethra but also from the epididymis indicates that the organism is a possible cause of epididymitis. The route of infection is not clear, but the ability of chlamydiae to infect columnar epithelial cells suggests that spread in continuity from the urethra is the most likely. Whether *C. trachomatis* acts alone or whether, as may happen in salpingitis, an initial chlamydial infection is then maintained by other organisms is not yet known. Epididymitis is a serious disease in its effects on fertility, and the possibility that in young men it may be a complication of chlamydial urethritis is clearly important.

Prostatitis

Acute bacterial prostatitis is usually caused by urinary tract pathogens such as *Esch. coli*. In the pre-antibiotic era *N. gonorrhoeae* was a common cause; the serious disease of that era is seldom seen today, although it is likely that some prostatic involvement still occurs in many infections of gonorrhoea. **Chronic bacterial prostatitis** is also usually caused by enterobacteria and is constantly associated with urinary tract infection, itself often secondary to structural disease. **Chronic abacterial prostatitis** is the least well understood entity. It is not associated with urinary tract infection, and its cause is uncertain. Some physicians, feeling perhaps that it is over diagnosed (which is almost certainly true) go so far as to deny its existence. It seems to us that this is too extreme a view, although it must be admitted that many patients with this diagnosis are really suffering from other disorders such as relapsing NGU or genital neurosis.

Patients with chronic abacterial prostatitis complain of perigenital discomfort, dysuria, intermittent urethral discharge, attacks of frequency of micturition and sometimes of painful orgasm. The prostate may feel enlarged, tender or oedematous ('boggy'), although these signs are not easy to elicit or interpret. The expressed prostatic fluid contains an excess of PMN (15 per mean field at a magnification × 400 is usually taken as diagnostic), but cultures on conventional media yield no growth. Because the disease has been regarded as infective there has been speculation that *C. trachomatis* might be involved in its pathogenesis. So far there is little evidence that this is so. Mårdh *et al.* (1978) studied a group of 53 men with non-acute prostatitis by culture and serology. *C. trachomatis* was recovered from the urethra of one patient, but not from any of 28 specimens of prostatic fluid. Six men showed, with immunofluorescence serology, IgG ⩾64 or IgM ⩾8. It was concluded that *C. trachomatis* played little or no part in chronic prostatitis.

It has been suggested (Ballard *et al.*, 1979) that chronic abacterial prostatitis may in some cases be the result of delayed hypersensitivity to *C. trachomatis*, by analogy with trachoma, some of whose manifestations may be the result of immune reactions to chlamydiae (Grayston and Wang, 1975). Support for this concept of prostatitis is at present only anecdotal.

Comment

We have occasionally recovered *C. trachomatis* from prostatic fluid, but it is difficult to be sure that the specimens are not contaminated by urethral material. Clinically, chronic abacterial prostatitis is a rather nebulous disease, and its aetiology remains uncertain. One might speculate that, as perhaps with salpingitis and epididymitis, an initial chlamydial infection of the prostate is continued by secondary invading organisms, but there is no evidence for or against this view at present.

Proctitis

The early investigators recovered chlamydiae from the rectum in women with chlamydial genital infection, and there seems to be no doubt that the organism can colonize this epithelium (Dunlop *et al.*, 1971b). In homosexual men rectal gonococcal infection is of major epidemiological importance, but there is little evidence that this is true of chlamydial infection. Goldmeier and Darougar (1977) obtained rectal isolates from two men with proctitis, in one of whom severe congestion and numerous follicles were seen with an operating microscope. Whether this is a common condition is not known, for the epidemiology of chlamydial infections in male homosexuals has not been studied to any great extent. Some workers have found urethral chlamydial infection to be uncommon in these men (see page 43) so the amount of chlamydial rectal infection in the homosexual population may not be great.

6

Genital tract infections in women

In the female genital tract *C. trachomatis* may infect the cervix, the urethra, the ducts of Bartholin's glands and the fallopian tubes. The organism is a possible cause of perihepatitis in women, and also infects the rectum.

Infection of the cervix

Cervical infection by *C. trachomatis* is common in women attending STD clinics. In the UK, isolation rates of 12–31 per cent have been reported (Table 6.1). In some clinics *C. trachomatis* is recovered from women more often than *N. gonorrhoeae* (Ridgway and Oriel, 1977).

Most chlamydial isolates come from acknowledged contacts of men with NGU; approximately one third of these women harbour chlamydiae (Hilton *et al.*, 1974; Oriel *et al.*, 1974; Rees *et al.*, 1977a). The difference in the isolation rates from contacts of men with *Chlamydia*-positive and *Chlamydia*-negative NGU is striking (Table 6.2); *C. trachomatis* is recovered from 45–68 per cent of contacts of culture-positive men, but from only 4–18 per cent of contacts of culture-negative men.

Cervical cultures for *C. trachomatis* have been performed on patients in family planning, gynaecology and other clinics which provide services for women (*see* Table 6.1). These heterogeneous clinics have populations which are not really comparable with each other, but it is clear that the isolation rates of *C. trachomatis* are low in comparison with those reported from STD clinics.

In view of the importance of neonatal chlamydial infection, the prevalence of chlamydiae during pregnancy is of particular interest, and this is shown in Table 6.3. The organisms may also be recovered in the immediate post-natal period. In Sweden, Mårdh *et al.*, (1980) recovered *C. trachomatis* from the cervix in 8 per cent of a group of puerperal women. It is to be expected that wide variations in the prevalence of chlamydial infections during pregnancy will occur, depending on the age, sexual activity and socio-economic status of the women.

Table 6.1 Recovery of *C. trachomatis* from cervical specimens from women attending STD and other clinics

Country	Authors	STD Clinics		Other Clinics		
		Number yielding chlamydiae/number examined	Percentage positive	Type of clinic	Number yielding chlamydiae/number examined	Percentage positive
UK	Hilton *et al.*, (1974)	86/279	31	Family planning	2/63	3
UK	Oriel *et al.*, (1974)	45/247	18			
UK	Hobson *et al.*, (1974)	38/190	20			
UK	Burns *et al.*, (1975)	76/638	12			
UK	Nayyar *et al.*, (1976)	60/300	20			
UK	Woolfitt and Watt, (1977)	53/200	26.5	Hospital staff	2/200	1
UK	Ridgway and Oriel, (1977)	269/1136	24			
UK	Oriel *et al.*, (1978)	58/284	20			
USA	Wentworth *et al.*, (1973)	83/385	22			
USA	Schachter *et al.*, (1975a)			Dysplasia drop in routine screening	23/665	3
USA	McCormack *et al.*, (1979)			Gynaecological O.P.	20/439	5
Finland	Paavonen *et al.*, (1978b)			Gynaecological O.P.	13/144	9
Sweden	Mårdh *et al.*, (1980)			Termination of pregnancy	14/231	16

Table 6.2 Recovery of *C. trachomatis* from cervix of contacts of men with Chlamydia-positive and Chlamydia-negative NGU

Country	Authors	Contacts of men with Chlamydia-positive NGU	Percentage positive	Contacts of men with Chlamydia-negative NGU	Percentage positive
		Number yielding chlamydiae/number tested			
UK	Oriel *et al.*, (1972)	12/18	67	1/23	4
UK	Alani *et al.*, (1977)	14/31	45	14/77	18
USA	Holmes *et al.*, (1975)	15/22	68	2/24	8
USA	Handsfield *et al.*, (1976)	15/24	63	1/21	5
Canada	Ghadirian and Robson, (1979)	7/11	64	1/10	10
Finland	Paavonen *et al.*, (1978a)	25/39	64	3/36	8
Finland	Terho, (1978b)	22/35	63	2/22	9

Table 6.3 Recovery of *C. trachomatis* from the cervix during pregnancy

Country	Authors	Stage of gestation (weeks)	Number yielding chlamydiae/number tested	Percentage positive
USA	Alexander *et al.*, (1977c)	36–40	18/142	13
USA	Schachter *et al.*, (1979c)	<16	36/900	4
USA	Frommell *et al.*, (1979)	<32	30/340	9
USA	Hammerschlag *et al.*, (1980)	12	Clinic 1 23/107	21.5
			Clinic 2 44/465	10
Sweden	Mårdh *et al.*, (1980)	8–13	14/231	6

Factors influencing isolation

Hormonal effects

It has been reported that the isolation rate of *C. trachomatis* is significantly higher in women who take oral contraceptives than in those who do not (Hilton *et al.*, 1974; Ripa *et al.*, 1978). Other workers have found no significant difference between the two groups in this respect (Burns *et al.*, 1975; Woolfitt and Watt, 1977; Oriel *et al.*, 1978). Tait *et al.* (1980) have suggested that a significant increase in the isolation rate is associated with oral contraception only in women who have a cervical erosion.

Hilton *et al.* (1974) found that all the chlamydial isolates obtained from a small group of pregnant women came from those in the last trimester of pregnancy, and suggested that the stage of pregnancy might influence the isolation rate; it was also suggested that isolation might be affected by the time of the menstrual cycle at which specimens were collected. Neither of these suggestions has been substantiated by other workers.

Associated infections

Multiple infections of the genital tract are common, and *C. trachomatis* may be associated with *N. gonorrhoeae*, mycoplasmas, Herpes simplex virus and other organisms (Wentworth *et al.*, 1973). In some cell culture systems the presence of *T. vaginalis* may sometimes make it impossible to recover chlamydiae from cervical specimens because of disruption of the cell monolayer, perhaps through overgrowth of *Streptococcus* spp.

The association of chlamydial and gonococcal infection of the cervix is common (Table 6.4). *C. trachomatis* is recovered from 27–63 per cent of women with gonorrhoea. The reason for this association is not clear, but since it is commoner in women than in men it seems likely that some women were already infected by chlamydiae before they contracted gonorrhoea (*see* page 102).

Serology

Serum antichlamydial antibodies are detected by micro-IF in 78–100 per cent of women yielding isolates of *C. trachomatis* from the cervix (Table 6.5). However, 31–87 per cent of culture-negative women are seropositive, so a single determination of antibodies does not necessarily indicate current infection. The prevalence of IgM antibodies is much lower; Schachter *et al.* (1979a) found serum IgM in 6 (32 per cent) of 19 culture-positive women and in 14 (19 per cent) of 74 culture-negative women. It has been difficult to demonstrate seroconversion or rising titres in women with chlamydial infection of the lower genital tract, partly because of high background levels of antibody and partly because many infections in women attending clinics are probably not of recent origin. The high antibody levels seen in isolation-negative women indicate previous exposure to *C. trachomatis*. The relationship between the prevalence of antibodies and increasing sexual experience has been neatly demonstrated by McCormack *et al.* (1979).

Symptoms and signs

There are no distinctive symptoms of genital chlamydial infection in women; approximately two thirds of those infected are symptomless (Burns *et al.*, 1975; Oriel *et al.*, 1978). When examined, about 20 per cent of women with confirmed chlamydial infection show a completely normal cervix (Hilton *et al.*, 1974; Oriel *et al.*, 1974; Rees *et al.*, 1977a). The remainder exhibit a variable amount of cervical discontinuity with or without a mucopurulent or purulent cervical exudate (Table 6.5). The terminology used to describe these changes has become rather confused, and there is much to be said for returning to the nomenclature of classical gynaecology (Jeffcoate, 1975). We will indicate the associations between chlamydial infection and cervical erosion, acute cervicitis and cervical microfollicles.

Cervical erosion

This is now often called cervical ectopy, which is probably a better term, but 'erosion' is more familiar and will be used here. It appears when the squamous

Table 6.4   Isolation of *C. trachomatis* from the cervix of women with gonorrhoea

Country	Authors	Number yielding chlamydiae/number tested	Percentage positive
UK	Oriel *et al.*, 1974	9/28	32
UK	Hilton *et al.*, 1974	36/57	63
UK	Nayyar *et al.*, 1976	18/66	27
UK	Burns *et al.*, 1975	14/32	44
UK	Ridgway and Oriel, 1977(a)	75/205	37
UK	Woolfitt and Watt, 1977	13/32	40
UK	Oriel *et al.*, 1978	15/48	31
UK	Davies *et al.*, 1978	111/210	53

Table 6.5   Relationship between serum antichlamydial antibodies and recovery of *C. trachomatis* from the cervix

Authors	Number of reactive sera (micro-IF titre $\geqslant 8$)/number tested			
	Isolation-positive	Percentage positive	Isolation-negative	Percentage positive
Richmond and Caul, (1977)	67/76	88	83/169	49
Oriel *et al.*, (1978)	40/51	78	64/207	31
Saikku and Paavonen, (1978)	55/58	95	61/91	67
Schachter *et al.*, (1979a)	34/34	100	121/139	87
Richmond *et al.*, (1980)	22/22	100	16/30	53

covering of the ectocervix is replaced by columnar epithelium, and is seen as a bright red area continuous with the endocervix, with a clearly defined outer edge. Cervical erosions are determined by the amounts of circulating oestrogen and progesterone (particularly the former). This is why they are commonly seen in neonates (from exposure to maternal oestrogen), during pregnancy, and in women taking an oral contraceptive. Erosions cannot be said to be a pathological state. Whether they are therefore normal is a matter of semantics, but since the distinction between erosion and no erosion is clinically valuable we have described the condition separately.

   C. trachomatis has been associated with cervical erosion by Schachter *et al.* (1975a) and by Burns *et al.* (1975). There is, of course, no suggestion that chlamydiae *cause* erosions, which are in any case unaffected by antibacterial therapy (Rees *et al.*, 1977a). Rather, it seems likely that an erosion simply presents a larger area of columnar epithelium for colonization by *C. trachomatis*.

Acute cervicitis

This is characterized by cervical congestion and erythema, with an abnormal cervical exudate. Acute cervicitis may supervene on a cervical erosion, in which case the erosion itself becomes congested and oedematous — the hypertrophic erosion of Rees *et al.*, (1977a). The best studies of the association of chlamydiae with these physical signs have come from the Liverpool group (Rees *et al.*, 1977a; Tait *et al.*, 1980). Their work shows that in contacts of men with NGU both hypertrophic erosion and endocervical mucopus are commoner in *Chlamydia*-positive than in *Chlamydia*-negative cases. If signs of cervicitis are narrowly defined as oedema of the areas covered by columnar epithelium and a mucopurulent endocervical exudate, there is a highly significant association between cervicitis and the presence of *C. trachomatis* (Tait *et al.*, 1980). After 3 weeks treatment with a tetracycline, most hypertrophic erosions reverted to simple erosions and mucopurulent cervical exudate became mucoid. In Sweden, Paavonen *et al.* (1978b) saw classical acute cervicitis in 8 (62 per cent) of 13 *Chlamydia*-positive, and in 43 (33 per cent) of 131 *Chlamydia*-negative, women.

The interpretation of these signs becomes much more difficult in less selected groups. Wentworth *et al.* (1973) found mixed infections with cervical pathogens to be commonplace; clearly, the more organisms are present the more difficult it becomes to attribute disease to any one of them. The problems of clinical diagnosis are aggravated by the difficulty which is encountered in practice of assigning a cervix to a diagnostic category; the appearance will depend on the state of the cervix before infection, on parity, on the use of contraceptive agents and devices, and on many other factors besides the presence of infecting agents. It is only when associated infection (particularly gonorrhoea and trichomoniasis) are excluded and restrictive criteria applied that associations between clinical cervicitis and *C. trachomatis* are seen. There is no doubt that chlamydiae can cause cervicitis. Indeed, Schachter and Dawson (1978) have described a prospective study in which the development of cervicitis, and its cure by tetracyclines, was seen in women following infection by *C. trachomatis*.

Cervical microfollicles
It has been suggested that these are diagnostic of chlamydial infection. Dunlop *et al.* (1966) first observed them with a colposcope in 18 (90 per cent) of 20 mothers of babies with inclusion conjunctivitis; presumably they are identical with the follicles described by the same group in association with chlamydial infections of the rectum and male urethra. In a later study Hare *et al.* (1980) examined a group of contacts of men with NGU; they recovered *C. trachomatis* from the cervix in 5 (45 per cent) of 11 women who had lymphocytic follicular cervicitis diagnosed by colposcopy and/or biopsy, but from only 1 (7 per cent) of 14 women without these changes.

Although expense and convenience limit the availability of colposcopy in most STD clinics, these microfollicles could be a useful clinical sign in special circumstances.

Histopathology

Cytoplasmic inclusions in epithelial cells are specifically related to chlamydial infection and were described many years ago. Braley (1938) examined cervical biopsy material from six mothers of babies with inclusion conjunctivitis, and reported inclusions confined to the zone of transitional epithelium. Using more advanced technology Swanson *et al.* (1975) examined biopsy specimens from two women with gonorrhoea and saw multiple vesicles within cervical epithelial cells; electron microscopy showed that these contained spherical bodies whose structure was typical of elementary bodies, reticulate bodies and intermediate forms of *C. trachomatis*. A marked inflammatory response was seen in subepithelial connective tissue, but these changes might have been due to gonococcal infection. One of the women yielded chlamydiae on cell culture.

Inclusions have also been identified in exfoliated cervical cells. Cervical cytology is widely available, and it is easy to see the attraction of using this test to diagnose chlamydial infection. This was attempted by Naib (1970), who identified intracytoplasmic inclusions in endocervical and parabasal cells in 33 (61 per cent) of 54 mothers of babies with neonatal inclusion conjunctivitis; there was also a marked inflammatory response, but this is difficult to assess since 42 of the women had trichomoniasis. Schachter and Dawson (1978) have expressed doubts on whether all the inclusions seen in this study were really chlamydial, and state that in their experience with Giemsa staining positive results were obtained in only 41 per cent of confirmed cervical chlamydial infections.

The other cellular responses to chlamydial infection are not pathognomonic. In chlamydial eye infections, conjunctival scrapings show epithelial cells with degenerative changes and an inflammatory exudate of PMN, lymphocytes, plasma cells and large mononuclear cells; this histological picture suggests, but does not prove, the diagnosis. Similar findings have been reported in cervical scrapings from the mothers of babies with neonatal inclusion conjunctivitis (Al-Hussaini, Jones and Dunlop, 1964).

Several workers, particularly in the UK, have commented on the association of *C. trachomatis* with inflammatory changes on cervical cytology, and it has been hinted that these changes could be used for diagnosis. The criteria are an increased number of parabasal cells, with evidence of reactive hyperplasia and atypical degenerative changes; the presence of excessive numbers of PMN may also be used in the assessment of inflammation (Wachtel, 1969). These changes are not, of course, specific to chlamydial infection, as they are present in association with other micro-organisms. In an early study we found 'inflammatory' cytology in 12 (46 per cent) of 26 *Chlamydia*-positive women, but this was also present in 48 (38 per cent) of 125 *Chlamydia*-negative women (Oriel *et al.*, 1974). Similar results have been reported by Paavonen *et al.*, (1978b): inflammatory changes were present in 69 per cent of culture-positive and in 42 per cent of culture-negative women. These differences are not however statistically significant. Burns *et al.* (1975) also found no difference between the two groups. It may be concluded that cytology is one of several markers of inflammation which may give positive results in chlamydial infection without being specifically related to it.

Comment

Some physicians feel tempted to equate cervicitis in women with urethritis in men. It is relatively easy to diagnose NGU, and it is suggested that its presumed counterpart in women, so-called 'non-specific genital infection', might also be diagnosed clinically. The process would be to establish the presence of cervicitis by clinical and laboratory examinations and to exclude

N. gonorrhoeae, T. vaginalis and Herpes simplex virus; a tentative diagnosis of chlamydial infection might thus be made, and the necessity of scarce and expensive laboratory procedures avoided.

It can be said at once that this idea is not practicable, and will lead to a correct diagnosis in only about half of cases (Oriel *et al.*, 1978). Over one third of women with a confirmed chlamydial infection show either a normal cervix or a simple erosion (Rees *et al.*, 1977a). Unless the criteria are restrictive, cervicitis is not an easy clinical diagnosis, and many cervices seen in clinical practice defy classification. Moreover cervicitis, however defined, has a complex pathogenesis involving multiple infecting agents, and even those infected by *C. trachomatis* may have associated infections.

The hard facts are that chlamydial infection of the cervix is a microbiological rather than a clinical diagnosis, and that without investigation by a valid laboratory procedure many infections will remain undiagnosed.

Persistence of cervical chlamydiae

The early workers sometimes noted that a succession of infants born to the same mother developed inclusion conjunctivitis, which suggested that cervical chlamydial infection could become chronic. Because of the pressure of re-infection it is not easy to substantiate this idea. Rees *et al.* (1977a) re-isolated *C. trachomatis* from 18 untreated women who were observed for up to 19 weeks, and in one case for 12 months. The best evidence for persistent infection comes from McCormack *et al.* (1979). Of 7 women with cervical chlamydial infection re-examined after 16–17 months, 4 were found still to be infected; 3 of the women denied intercourse since their first examination. These studies suggest that untreated chlamydial infections in women may persist for many months.

Cervical dysplasia

Little is known of the long term effects of cervical chlamydial infection. Its prevalence in women with cervical dysplasia was investigated by Schachter *et al.*, (1975b). The isolation rates were 4.1 per cent for women with dysplasia and 0.8 per cent in a cancer screening clinic. Using micro-IF serology, the authors found antichlamydial antibodies at titre ⩾16 in 43 per cent of women with dysplasia and in 25 per cent in the cancer screening clinic. However, these two populations were evidently not matched for age, parity, number of sex partners or past history of STD.

Paavonen *et al.* (1979a) reported broadly similar results. Using a single antigen IF test, they reported titres of ⩾64 in 41 per cent of patients with cervical atypia and in 20 per cent of a control group. Carr, Hanna and Jawetz (1979) reported an association between chlamydial infection as indicated by the presence of local antichlamydial antibodies and Papanicolaou Class 2 or 3 cytology. Isolation of *C. trachomatis* was not attempted. For the most part these local antibodies corresponded with serum antibodies, and they may not have been produced locally, or indicate current cervical infection (see page 33).

A high prevalence of antichlamydial antibodies is related to sexual activity and multiple partners, which is a well known epidemiological characteristic of women with cervical dysplasia. The available data are reminiscent of the early studies of cervical atypia in relation to Herpes virus simplex type 2 infections, and as in those studies adequate case controls are essential if an epidemiological correlation of dysplasia and infection is sought. Specific associations between *C. trachomatis* infections and dysplasia cannot be determined from present evidence.

Salpingitis

Salpingitis is an important disease. Apart from the immediate morbidity, subsequent tubal occlusion may cause infertility and an increased risk of ectopic gestation. The early workers noted salpingitis in some mothers whose babies had inclusion conjunctivitis (Dunlop *et al.*, 1966), and salpingitis is not infrequently seen in association with cervical chlamydial infection. Rees *et al.* (1977a) have stressed the importance of salpingitis associated with *C. trachomatis* during the puerperium.

During the past five years interest in the role of *C. trachomatis* in pelvic inflammatory disease (PID) has increased. In part this is because laparoscopy is now widely available, and while its use for diagnosis in salpingitis is not generally agreed among gynaecologists, some workers have been able to collect specimens for microbiology directly from the tubes with this technique. Tubal specimens are more valuable than cervical specimens in determining the aetiology of salpingitis. The recovery of *C. trachomatis* from the cervix provides only suggestive evidence that this organism is involved in the pathogenesis of salpingitis, although it must be remembered that in many cases of gonococcal salpingitis *N. gonorrhoeae* has been recovered only from the cervix and not from the fallopian tubes (Sweet *et al.*, 1980). In addition to isolation studies, serology with the micro-IF technique has been used to investigate the role of *C. trachomatis* in PID by demonstrating high IgG levels, rising antibody titres and the presence of IgM antibody in some women with the disease.

The results of attempts to recover *C. trachomatis* from women with salpingitis are summarized in Table 6.6. The most convincing findings have come from the workers at Lund, in Sweden, who have studied salpingitis systematically for many years. Mårdh *et al.* (1977) investigated a group of women with laparoscopically confirmed salpingitis. *C. trachomatis* was isolated from the cervix in 19 (36 per cent) of 53 women and from the fallopian tubes in 6 (30 per cent) of 20 women (3 from swabs and 3 from small biopsy specimens). No isolates were obtained from cervical and tubal specimens in control groups of women without salpingitis. Cervical cultures for *N. gonorrhoeae* were positive in 5 (9 per cent) of the 53 women with salpingitis, but all tubal cultures for this organism were negative.

Paavonen *et al.*, (1979c) recovered *C. trachomatis* from the cervix and/or urethra in 27 (26 per cent) of 106 women with acute salpingitis. Rising titres of antichlamydial antibody were found in 10 (48 per cent) of 22 isolation-positive women and in 9 (18 per cent) of 50 isolation-negative women. The GMT of IgG antibodies in the salpingitis group was 219 if *C. trachomatis* was isolated and 73 if it was not; in symptomless isolation-negative women the GMT was 80.

Table 6.6 Isolation of C. trachomatis from the cervix and the fallopian tubes of women with salpingitis and women without salpingitis

Authors	Salpingitis confirmed by laparoscopy	Number yielding chlamydiae/number tested							
		Cervix				Fallopian tubes			
		Women with salpingitis	Percentage positive	Controls	Percentage positive	Women with salpingitis	Percentage positive	Controls	Percentage positive
Eschenbach et al., (1975)	No	10/49	20	43/200	21.5				
Hamark et al., (1976)	Yes	6/21	29			1/21	5		
Mårdh et al., (1977)	Yes	19/53	36	0/12	0	6/20	30	0/5	0
Paavonen et al., (1979c)	No	27/106	26						

Simmons *et al.* (1979) studied the role of *C. trachomatis* in PID which had been diagnosed without laparoscopy by performing single measurements of IgG and IgM antibody in these patients and in women with uncomplicated lower genital tract infections. They accepted a level of ≥64 for IgG and ≥8 for IgM antichlamydial antibody as suggestive of active chlamydial infection. In women with PID defined by strict criteria there were significantly higher levels of IgG (but not IgM) antibodies than in women with lower genital tract infections. In a subsequent study Treharne *et al.* (1979) applied the same techniques to 143 women with laparoscopically confirmed PID and to 19 women without genital tract infection. In the PID group, 62 per cent had IgG antichlamydial antibody levels of ≥64, but these levels were only present in 10.5 per cent of controls. There was a correlation between the severity of salpingitis and the GMT of IgG antibody. IgM antibodies, on the other hand, were present at a level of ≥8 in only 23 per cent of women with salpingitis and in 5 per cent of controls.

A convincing demonstration of active chlamydial infection in salpingitis is provided by Møller *et al.*, (1979). Two fallopian tubes which had been excised from two women with acute salpingitis were available for examination *C. trachomatis* was isolated from one specimen and inclusions were seen in the other. In both patients there had been a significant change in micro-IF antibodies to *C. trachomatis* during the course of their disease. The first showed an IgM titre of 128 and a threefold rise of titre of IgG antibody. The second showed no IgM antibodies, but a significant fall in IgG titre occured during convalescence. Histological examination of both tubes showed acute inflammatory changes through all layers, resembling the changes seen in the tubes of patients with gonococcal salpingitis.

Discussion

There can be no doubt that *C. trachomatis* is involved in the pathogenesis of PID. The isolation studies show that in some parts of the world chlamydiae are recovered from inflamed fallopian tubes more often than *N. gonorrhoeae*. The serological data support the importance of *C. trachomatis* in the aetiology of PID. Since serology alone cannot differentiate chlamydial infection of the fallopian tubes from infection of the lower genital tract, caution should be used both in applying the technique for diagnostic purposes and for making quantitative estimates of the role of *C. trachomatis* in PID.

The pathological processes involved in chlamydial salpingitis are not clearly understood. Experimental infection of grivet monkeys with *C. trachomatis* indicates that the organism causes salpingitis by canalicular spread from the lower genital tract (Møller and Mårdh, 1980); this is the way in which gonococcal infection of the fallopian tubes is believed to occur (Falk, 1946).

In organ culture of human fallopian tubes, gonococci infect tubal mucosa and invade and destroy epithelial cells (Ward, Watt and Robertson, 1974). This technique has been used to study the effects of *C. trachomatis* infection (Hutchinson, Taylor-Robinson and Dourmashkin, 1979). Although the organisms replicated in the tissues, no evidence of extensive epithelial damage was observed, and there was no loss of ciliary activity. Thus in this system *C.*

trachomatis appears to be less pathogenic than *N. gonorrhoeae*. There are two ways of reconciling these findings with the concept that *C. trachomatis* causes salpingitis. The first is that the disease represents an immunological response of the host to chlamydial infection; the second, that clinical disease occurs as the result of combined infection with chlamydiae and other micro-organisms. It is interesting to note that both of these suggestions have been made in connection with the pathogenesis of trachoma.

The microbiology of PID is complex, and is very unlikely to be uniform throughout the world. In some countries *C. trachomatis* is of prime importance in aetiology, but it would be very unwise to extrapolate this to other areas without supporting evidence. In many localities *N. gonorrhoeae* maintains its traditional role as a major cause of PID. This is true in San Francisco for example, as the recent data of Sweet *et al.* (1980) indicate; these workers found little evidence of involvement of *C. trachomatis* in the pathogenesis of PID in their patients. Further studies in other countries are obviously needed.

Perihepatitis

Acute perihepatitis (the Fitz-Hugh-Curtis syndrome) is characterized by the development of right-sided upper abdominal pain, usually of sudden onset, with accompanying tenderness in the right upper quadrant. In its early stages there is localized peritonitis over the peritoneal covering of the anterior surface of the liver and adjacent abdominal wall; later, 'violin-string' adhesions may develop. Liver function tests may or may not be abnormal.

Although the syndrome is best known as a complication of gonococcal salpingitis, it has been suggested that it may also be caused by *C. trachomatis*. Müller-Schoop *et al.*, (1978) studied 11 young women with acute peritonitis, confirmed by laparoscopy, of whom 7 also had symptoms suggesting peri-hepatitis — pain and tenderness in the right upper quadrant and abnormal liver function tests. Of these 11 patients, 9 had serological evidence of active chlamydial infection; 4 of the women also had gonorrhoea. More recently, Wølner-Hanssen, Weström and Mårdh (1980) have described 3 patients with acute perihepatitis verified by laparoscopy or laparotomy. Although *C. trachomatis* was not recovered from the inflamed peritoneal surfaces, there was evidence of current chlamydial infection from positive cervical cultures or from serology. We have seen a similar case presenting in the puerperium in the mother of a baby with neonatal inclusion conjunctivitis. Acute right-sided upper abdominal pain may thus be an occasional presentation of genital chlamydial infection.

Infection of other sites

Bartholin's ducts

Davies *et al.*, (1978) isolated chlamydiae from Bartholin's ducts in 9 women, of whom 7 had concurrent gonorrhoea. Contamination of specimens by chlamydiae from other genital sites is possible, but seems unlikely from the data. *N. gonorrhoeae* infects Bartholin's glands and their ducts, and it would not be surprising if *C. trachomatis* behaved similarly, or if double infections occurred.

Urethra

There is evidence which suggests that *C. trachomatis*, like *N. gonorrhoeae*, may infect the female urethra as well as the cervix. The isolation of chlamydiae from the urethra of a woman was first reported by Dunlop, *et al.* (1972). The patient complained of recurrent dysuria and frequency of micturition, and she also had a cervical chlamydial infection. Subsequently, other workers reported urethral isolates of *C. trachomatis* from NGU contacts and from women with chlamydial eye infections. In these early studies it was unusual to isolate chlamydiae from the urethra without simultaneous isolates from the cervix (Oriel *et al.*, 1972), and it was obviously possible that the urethral 'isolates' were due to contamination. However, Woolfitt and Watt (1977) found that in a group of 53 women who yielded *C. trachomatis* from the urogenital tract, isolates were obtained from the cervix alone in 32, from the cervix and urethra in 16, and from the urethra alone in 5 patients, which suggests that urethral chlamydial infection may not be infrequent.

Paavonen (1979) related the isolation of *C. trachomatis* to urinary symptoms in a group of 99 NGU contacts. He obtained a striking isolation rate from the urethra, for chlamydiae were recovered from the cervix in 28 women, from the cervix and urethra in 46, and from the urethra alone in 25. While dysuria and frequency of micturition were described by 54 per cent of women with positive urethral cultures, they were present in only 21 per cent of women with infection confined to the cervix. These results renewed interest in an old idea – that *C. trachomatis* might be related in some way to the 'urethral syndrome'.

The 'urethral syndrome' is characterized by attacks of dysuria and frequency of micturition without significant bacteriuria; its pathogenesis is a mystery, and treatment notoriously unsatisfactory. Stamm *et al.* (1980) have performed a prospective study in a group of 16 women with the syndrome who had pyuria. They found evidence of current chlamydial infection in 10 of them — 7 yielded chlamydiae from the urethra and/or cervix, and 3 were culture-negative but showed a fourfold rise or fall of micro-IF antibody titre. Only 1 of 16 women with the urethral syndrome without pyuria showed evidence of chlamydial infection. Patients with the 'urethral syndrome' associated with chlamydial infection acknowledged a recent change of sex partner more often than women with dysuria and frequency of micturition due to other organisms such as coliforms or staphylococci.

Comment

As with other diseases newly associated with *C. trachomatis*, the evidence that the urethral syndrome is related to *C. trachomatis* is intriguing and suggestive, but not conclusive. The investigations of Stamm *et al.* (1980) show the way in which research in this area can usefully be pursued, but there will obviously be problems in assembling a reasonably large group of women for study who satisfy the criteria of the 'urethral syndrome' before they are treated with antibiotics. However, it is already clear that urethral chlamydial infection in women may cause otherwise unexplained dysuria, and culture from the female urethra may be a useful diagnostic procedure in these patients.

Rectum

Associated rectal and genital infections by *C. trachomatis* in women have been demonstrated. Dunlop *et al.*, (1971b) studied a group of 82 women with chlamydial infection; isolates were obtained from the genital tract alone in 15 patients, from the genital tract and rectum in 12 and from the rectum alone in one. Isolates were associated with mucosal changes visible with the operating microscope in 5 of 13 women with rectal infections; follicles, 'cobblestones', scarring and congestion were seen. In 5 more patients with chlamydial rectal infection the rectal mucosa was normal but a mucopurulent exudate was seen. Of 69 culture-negative patients mucosal changes were seen in 4 and a mucopurulent exudate in 7.

Little interest has been shown in rectal chlamydial infection in women, but the work of the London Hospital group suggests that it may be quite common. Whether there is any clinical benefit to be derived from investigating this area as well as the genital tract is not yet clear.

Infertility, abortion and fetal death

Epididymitis and salpingitis may both be followed by infertility, and the role of *C. trachomatis* in these diseases has already been discussed (*see* pages 50 and 61). Whether chlamydial infection of the female genital tract which is not causing tubal occlusion can cause infertility is not clear. Paavonen *et al.*, (1979b) recovered *C. trachomatis* from the cervix of 10 (20 per cent) of 51 women without occlusion who were being investigated for infertility; the prevalence of chlamydiae in their general gynaecological population was 9 per cent. This suggests that the relationship between chlamydial infection and infertility might be worth investigating. However, in a pilot study we have failed to recover *C. trachomatis* from the cervix or fallopian tubes of women with non-occlusive infertility (Kelsey, Lachelin and Ridgway, unpublished data); furthermore, it will be remembered that doxycycline (active against *C. trachomatis*) has failed to improve fertility when given empirically to couples with non-occlusive infertility (Harrison, de Louvois and Blades, 1975). Present evidence does not allow any conclusion to be drawn on the role (if any) of *C. trachomatis* in infertility.

In some animals, such as sheep, *C. psittaci* is a definite cause of abortion, but it is not yet known whether *C. trachomatis* has this effect in humans. Schachter (1967) isolated chlamydiae from 4 of 22 abortion specimens, but the subject has received little further attention so far. *C. trachomatis* infection may, however, be related to fetal morbidity. In a prospective study of *Chlamydia* infection in pregnancy Martin *et al.*, (1979) noted that fetal death occurred in 6 (30 per cent) of 20 culture-positive women as compared with 18 (11 per cent) of 164 culture-negative women; 4 of 6 women whose fetuses died had endometritis, amnionitis or salpingitis. If chlamydial infection during pregnancy is a significant cause of fetal death, the high prevalence of infection in some ante-natal populations must be viewed with concern. There can be no doubt that *C. trachomatis*, like *N. gonorrhoeae*, poses a major and continuing threat to the health and welfare of women.

7

Neonatal infection

A baby born through a maternal genital tract infected by *C. trachomatis* may, during the first few weeks of life, become colonized by the organism. The sites from which chlamydiae have been recovered during this period are shown below:

Conjunctiva

Nasopharynx
Middle ear (Myringotomy)
Trachea

Lung (Biopsy)

Rectum

Vagina

In some of these, for example the eye, the organism is often associated with clinical disease; in others, such as the pharynx or rectum, there is no apparent disease and the significance of colonization is uncertain. Within the last few years the number of neonatal syndromes thought to be the result of chlamydial infection has increased considerably.

Infection of the eye

Precise figures for the incidence of chlamydial eye infection in neonates in the UK are not available, but it is certainly commoner than gonococcal ophthalmia. In a selected group of 103 babies with neonatal conjunctivitis examined in Liverpool, *N. gonorrhoeae* was isolated from 11 and *C. trachomatis* from 33 (Rees *et al.*, 1977b); in London, chlamydial ophthalmia neonatorum is said to be at least five times as common as the gonococcal form (Dunlop, 1975). In a clinic in San Francisco with a 4 per cent isolation rate of *C. trachomatis* from the cervix in pregnant women, Schachter *et al.* (1979c) estimate 14 cases of chlamydial conjunctivitis per 1000 live births.

Neonatal inclusion conjunctivitis (inclusion blennorrhoea) appears in most infants between the 3rd and the 13th day of life (Rees *et al.*, 1977b). A wide range of clinical disease is seen, varying between mild conjunctivitis ('sticky eye') to severe inflammation. The disease is described on page 38.

Infection of the upper respiratory tract

In a study of a group of babies with inclusion conjunctivitis, Freedman *et al.* (1966) commented on the frequent occurrence of mucopurulent rhinitis, and *C. trachomatis* was recovered from the nasal secretions of some of the infants. Colonization of the nasopharynx by chlamydiae is not necessarily associated with clinical evidence of infection; the organisms have been recovered from the nasopharynx in infants with inclusion conjunctivitis and no respiratory disease (Beem and Saxon, 1977), or indeed from infants without any apparent respiratory and eye disease (Schachter *et al.*, 1979b).

Infection of the middle ear may follow pharyngeal infection by respiratory tract pathogens, and it would not be surprising if this occurred with *C. trachomatis*. Otitis media has been noticed in adults with chlamydial eye infections, and *C. trachomatis* has been recovered from fluid obtained by myringotomy from one of these patients (Dawson and Schachter, 1967). There is thus reasonable evidence that *C. trachomatis* may cause otitis media in some circumstances. Evidence that the organism may cause secretory otitis media in neonates has come from the studies of Tipple, Beem and Saxon (1979) into chlamydial pneumonia in infants. They examined one or both tympanic membranes in 37 *Chlamydia*-positive infants and found evidence of middle ear abnormalities in more than half of them. Myringotomies performed on 11 of these patients yielded gelatinous material, and *C. trachomatis* was recovered from 3 of the ear aspirates. These findings suggest that secretory otitis media occurs in infants with chlamydial infection of the respiratory tract; its pathogenesis and clinical importance await definition.

Pneumonia

The importance of *C. trachomatis* in neonatal disease was emphasized when it was reported that respiratory tract colonization with the organism may be associated with a distinctive afebrile pneumonia syndrome. Schachter *et al.* (1975c) described an infant in whom pneumonia had followed inclusion conjunctivitis; *C. trachomatis* was recovered from the sputum at a time when conjunctival cultures were sterile.Beem and Saxon (1977) defined the clinical characteristics of this respiratory disease and subsequently expanded their study group to 41 infants (Tipple, Beem and Saxon, 1979). Other cases of the disease in North America have also been described by Harrison *et al.* (1978) and Embil, Ozere and MacDonald, (1978), and in Israel by Sagy *et al.* (1980).

The pneumonia syndrome is an afebrile and relatively non-toxic illness, presenting between the 4th and 12th weeks of life. Partial nasal obstruction with mucoid discharge is often present, together with otitis media (*see* above), but the predominating features are tachypnoea and a distinctive staccato paroxysmal cough. Chest radiography shows hyperexpansion, with bilateral symmetrical diffuse interstitial and patchy alveolar infiltrates. Laboratory investigation shows consistently raised IgA, IgM and IgG, and sometimes eosinophilia. *C. trachomatis* is recovered from nasopharyngeal or tracheal specimens. Very high antichlamydial IgG titres are present — higher than are seen in any other *Chlamydia*-associated disease, and IgM antibodies are also present in some patients. The disease runs a protracted course with eventual recovery, and the prognosis for life is apparently good, although a life-threatening illness in an infant of two weeks has been described by Sagy *et al.* (1980). Nothing is known of the prognosis of unrecognized and untreated *Chlamydia*-associated pneumonia.

The relationship between the pneumonia syndrome and antecedent conjunctival infection is not completely clear. In about half of infants with the syndrome there is no history or clinical evidence of eye infection, and conjunctival cultures for *C. trachomatis* are negative (Beem and Saxon, 1977; Harrison *et al.*, 1978). On the other hand, a high prevalence of tear antibodies in these babies suggests that apparent or inapparent conjunctival infection is usual before the onset of pneumonia (Harrison, *et al.*, 1978).

The association between *C. trachomatis* and this pneumonia syndrome was strengthened when chlamydiae were recovered from lung tissue obtained from an affected baby by open biopsy (Frommell, Bruhn and Schwartzman, 1977). Their patient also had a cytomegalovirus infection, and it was argued at the time that this organism might have caused the pneumonia either alone or in combination with *C. trachomatis*. However, the second lung biopsy to yield chlamydiae (Arth *et al.*, 1978) was from a baby without mixed infection; the histology of the specimen showed pleural congestion, almost total alveolar consolidation and partial bronchial consolidation, with eosinophils, granular pneumocytes and focal aggregates of neutrophils.

Comment

What is the evidence that *C. trachomatis* actually causes this pneumonia syndrome, rather than being an accidental contaminant? In summary, the agent is recovered from more infants with the syndrome than from control infants from the same population; there are significantly higher titres of antichlamydial antibodies in cases than in controls; and clinical improvement following treatment with antimicrobial agents which are active against *C. trachomatis* is accompanied by disappearance of demonstrable chlamydiae. This evidence is supported by the results of inoculation of the respiratory tract of three infant baboons with a strain of *C. trachomatis* from a human infant with pneumonia (Harrison *et al.*, 1979). One animal showed a persistent nasopharyngeal chlamydial infection, radiological evidence of pneumonia, and histological changes almost identical to those seen in the human neonatal pneumonia syndrome. The second and third animals also maintained nasopharyngeal carriage of the organisms; one of them had a patchy pneumonitis at autopsy. Despite the evidence reviewed above, there are some problems which require clarification. Of Tipple, Beem and Saxon's final group of 41 infants with *Chlamydia*-associated pneumonia, 18 (44 per cent) were also infected by one or more viruses; while it seems unlikely from the data that these were responsible for the clinical illness, the possibility of a synergistic effect, as the authors themselves point out, has not been excluded. The age of onset, too, is puzzling. Neonatal inclusion conjunctivitis usually appears within the first two weeks of life, but the pneumonia syndrome is delayed until the second month. How can this be explained? It could be postulated that pulmonary infection develops slowly, or is delayed by antibody reactions, but it is also possible that hypersensitivity is a major factor. This second idea is attractive, and would also explain the eosinophilia which is often present; the very high titres of antibody might then be due to immunological over-reaction.

Nearly all the reports of the neonatal pneumonia syndrome have come from North America, and it is clear that some of the series of patients are from selected population groups; thus Beem and Saxon's (1977) patients were predominantly from a black inner city area, and Harrison *et al.* (1978) found that the syndrome was particularly associated with mothers who were young, single and in lower socio-economic groups. It may be that these populations are heavily exposed to *Chlamydia*, but in other areas where there is much genital chlamydial infection and neonatal eye disease, for example in Liverpool, the pneumonia syndrome is apparently very rare (Hobson and Rees, 1977). One explanation of this phenomenon might be the different arrangements for primary medical care of babies which exist in the UK and in the USA. In the former, this is delivered by general practitioners, and it is probable that an afebrile and non-toxic infant with paroxysmal cough would be treated with antibiotics without extensive investigation. In the USA, on the other hand, and particularly in the lower socio-economic groups mentioned above, primary care is delivered by hospital-based paediatricians, and the radiological and biochemical changes associated with the pneumonia syndrome might be more readily detected. Nevertheless, it would be surprising if clinical reports of cases of the syndrome did not soon appear from the UK and other European countries.

Infection of other sites

Vaginal colonization by *C. trachomatis* in the absence of clinical disease has been recorded in neonates, and is presumed to be due to external contamination during birth (Schachter *et al.*, 1979b). Isolates of the organisms from the rectum have also been recorded in infants born to infected mothers. Positive cultures from this site recorded by Schachter *et al.* (1979b) included two from babies with the pneumonia syndrome which were the only positive cultures obtained from these patients. Sampling from this site may well be of value to the clinician in investigating babies for chlamydial disease.

Prospective studies show that chlamydiae are not recovered from the rectum until the 6th–12th week of life, so this infection may not be directly acquired during birth, but rather due to ingestion of organisms derived from ocular or upper respiratory infections. Tipple, Beem and Saxon (1979) noted poor weight gain in some infants with the pneumonia syndrome prior to the onset of chest disease; while this was not shown to be specifically related to the recovery of chlamydiae from the rectum, the possibility of infection of the intestinal epithelium will require active consideration.

Prematurity

Rees *et al.*, (1977b) noted gestation periods of 30–37 weeks in 12 (41 per cent) of 29 babies with neonatal inclusion conjunctivitis; two babies had ventricular septal defects. Prematurity may be due to chlamydial infection of the membranes overlying the internal os causing their premature rupture; this phenomenon, if it occurs, could be related to the fetal loss in infected mothers which has already been described (see page 66). However the pathogenesis of *Chlamydia*-associated prematurity is speculative; indeed, it is uncertain whether it is a real clinical entity.

Natural history of neonatal chlamydial infection

The expansion of the clinical spectrum of neonatal chlamydial infection has prompted a series of prospective studies of pregnant women with cervical chlamydial infection who were left untreated in order to define the risks to the babies in these circumstances. These are summarized in Table 7.1.

The results indicate that between 22–60 per cent of infants exposed to maternal chlamydial infection during birth will develop chlamydial eye disease. The risk of pneumonia is between one half and one quarter of the risk of ophthalmia. Clearly, some babies develop the pneumonia syndrome with no antecedent history or clinical evidence of eye infection. Conversely, shedding of chlamydiae from the upper respiratory tract in babies with or without eye infection may occur without any apparent respiratory disease.

A reasonable hypothesis is that chlamydial infection of the eye, nasopharynx and perhaps the vagina occurs soon after birth through direct exposure to the organisms during delivery. Pneumonia, through a mechanism which is not yet clear, occurs some weeks later in a proportion of these infants. The route and significance of rectal colonization is unknown.

Nothing is known about the long term effects, if any, of untreated chlamydial infection of the respiratory or gastro-intestinal tracts in infancy. If these occurred, they would add to the importance of perinatal chlamydial infection. Even now, though, the range and prevalence of neonatal disease is such as to cause anxiety, and the question of prophylaxis, either by identifying and treating infected women during pregnancy or by measures adopted at or soon after birth, requires active consideration. Some of these problems will be considered again in a later chapter (see page 109).

Table 7.1 Incidence of conjunctival infection and pneumonia in infants born to mothers with cervical infection by *C. trachomatis*

Country	Authors	Number of infants studied	Maximum duration of observation (months)	Conjunctival infection		Pneumonia	
				Clinical	Attributed to *C. trachomatis*	Clinical	Attributed to *C. trachomatis*
USA	Alexander et al., (1977)	18	3	9	6	5	4
USA	Schachter et al., (1979c)	20	12	13	7	2	2
USA	Frommell et al., (1979)	18	9	8	8	1	1
USA	Hammerschlag et al., (1979)	6	6	2	2		

8

Miscellaneous diseases

Reiter's syndrome

This potentially chronic and disabling disease usually follows a clinically apparent infection. On the continent of Europe and in North Africa and Asia this infection is usually dysenteric, but in the UK and North America it is a sexually acquired urethritis. The classical triad of manifestations of Reiter's syndrome is urethritis, conjunctivitis and arthritis, but today it is defined in terms of three of the following; urethritis/prostatitis, arthritis, conjunctivitis/uveitis, circinate balanitis/keratoderma blenorrhagica. It is not clear whether sexually acquired reactive arthritis (Keat *et al.*, 1978) is a *forme fruste* of the same disease. Reiter's syndrome is much commoner in men than in women, and often runs a chronic and relapsing course. Clinical experience has shown that although the urethritis will improve with antibiotics these drugs do not appear to affect the other components of the syndrome, nor do they reduce the liability to recurrences.

Reiter's syndrome was first linked with *C. trachomatis* two decades ago, when inclusions were seen in urethral specimens from a man with the disease (Siboulet and Galistin, 1962). Subsequent evidence of a possible connection came from both isolation studies and serology. Several workers in Western Europe and the USA have reported the results of urethral culture for *C. trachomatis* in men with Reiter's syndrome (Table 8.1). Although none of these investigations was controlled, the isolation rates, while lower than in unselected cases of NGU, are higher than in men without urethritis.

The serological evidence for the involvement of *C. trachomatis* in Reiter's syndrome is again beset by the problem of controls. In the published studies control groups have come from both venereal disease and rheumatology clinics: it is not clear which of these provide the best matched controls. The first studies, which used complement fixation tests, are summarized in Table 8.2. It is difficult to decide what these results mean. Evidence of active infection from complement fixation tests normally requires either a rising titre or seroconversion; a single titre estimation is of questionable significance. In fact, most of the data show little difference between patients with Reiter's

Table 8.1   Isolation of *C. trachomatis* from the urethra of men with Reiter's syndrome

Author	Number yielding chlamydiae/number tested	Percentage positive
Vaughan-Jackson *et al.*, (1972)	3/10	30
Gordon *et al.*, (1973)	1/16	6
Schachter, (1976)	12/81	15
Kousa *et al.*, (1978)	40/103	39

Table 8.2   Complement fixing antibody titres against chlamydial group antigen in patients with Reiter's syndrome and controls

Authors	Patients with Reiter's syndrome		controls		
	Number with titres ≥16/number tested	Percentage seropositive	Source	Number with titres ≥16/number tested	Percentage seropositive
Sharp, Lidsky and Riley, (1968)	1/7	14	STD clinic	8/56	14
Kinsella, Norton and Ziff, (1968)	9/24	37	STD clinic	61/168	36
			Patients with ankylosing spondylitis	0/46	0
Ford, (1968)	14/50	28	STD clinic	15/100	15
Schachter, (1971)	18/24	21	STD clinic	78/1000	8
			Men with NGU	6/163	4
			Patients in arthritis clinic	60/2000	3
Vaughan-Jackson *et al.*, (1972)	0/25	0			
Kousa *et al.*, (1978)	24/104	23			

syndrome than in matched control subjects. Whether these complement fixing antibodies indicate urethral infection by *C. trachomatis* or systemic chlamydial disease is not clear.

The micro-IF test has also been used. Vaughan-Jackson *et al.* (1972) found titres of ≥8 in 80 per cent, and Kousa *et al.* (1978) in 87 per cent, of patients with Reiter's syndrome, but neither series was adequately controlled. Keat *et al.* (1980) have found higher levels of antichlamydial antibodies by micro-IF in sexually acquired reactive arthritis than in NGU, and have observed an increase in antibody titres during periods of active joint disease.

Comment

The data associating *C. trachomatis* with Reiter's syndrome, although not compelling, cannot be dismissed. How is it to be interpreted? *C. trachomatis* cannot be the only cause of the disease, because a substantial number of cases are post-dysenteric rather than post-urethritic. It seems unlikely that Reiter's syndrome is due to direct infection of joints. Although Schachter *et al.* (1966) reported chlamydial isolates from synovial fluid, synovial membrane and the conjunctivae of patients with Reiter's syndrome, others have failed to recover chlamydiae from the synovial fluid of affected joints (Vaughan-Jackson *et al.*, 1972; Mårdh, 1975). Furthermore, the arthritis and the skin and ocular manifestations are uninfluenced by antibiotics.

It seems far more probable that Reiter's syndrome is determined immunologically. In this regard the high association of a single histocompatability antigen, HLA B-27, with Reiter's syndrome as first reported by Brewerton *et al.* (1973) is especially important. It may be that *C. trachomatis* is one of several infective agents which will precipitate Reiter's syndrome in a genetically predisposed individual. The mechanism is not clear, but it is conceivable that dissemination of chlamydial antigen from the genital site is followed by local immune responses which determine the clinical signs.

Gastro-intestinal disease

The rectum is one of the sites from which *C. trachomatis* has been recovered in neonates (page 66). Whether the organisms infect other parts of the gastro-intestinal tract in infants, and if so whether such infection causes disease, is unknown.

The possibility that chlamydiae might determine intestinal disease in adults was raised when Schuller *et al.* (1979) reported a significant association of chlamydial antibodies detected by immunofluorescence in patients with Crohn's disease in comparison with patients with other gastro-intestinal diseases. However, this association has not been confirmed by three other groups (Taylor-Robinson *et al.*, 1979; Munro *et al.*, 1979; Swarbrick *et al.*, 1979).

Endocarditis

Endocarditis caused by *C. psittaci* has been recorded several times, but recently a case of endocarditis apparently due to infection with *C. trachomatis* immunotype F has been reported (Van der Bel Kahn *et al.*, 1978). The patient was a 25-year-old woman in the 30th week of pregnancy who presented with a fulminating febrile illness which quickly proved fatal. At necropsy vegetations were seen on the aortic valve, and electron microscopy of these showed structures which resembled chlamydial elementary bodies. A retrospective analysis of serum samples by micro-IF showed a 32-fold rise in IgM antibody and a 16-fold rise in IgG antibody to immunotype F. The pathological evidence indicates recent infection, but the source of this, and the natural history of the infection, cannot now be determined.

Pharyngeal infection

C. trachomatis can colonise the pharynx, as it has been recovered from this area in patients with inclusion conjunctivitis (Dawson and Schachter, 1967). By analogy with gonorrhoea, where pharyngeal infection correlates with a history of fellatio, it might be thought that pharyngeal infection with chlamydiae could occur in the same way. Schachter and Atwood (1975) described a woman with symptomatic pharyngitis who yielded *C. trachomatis* on culture; she had had fellatio with a man with recurrent NGU before her symptoms began. The data of Bowie, Alexander and Holmes (1977) shows that this sort of infection is probably a rare event. These workers took pharyngeal swabs from 117 women who admitted fellatio with men with NGU (11 of the men were known to have chlamydial urethritis), but they failed to obtain a single isolate.

Lower respiratory tract infection

C. trachomatis acquired during birth can invade the respiratory tract in infants and induce pneumonia (*see* page 69). It has recently been suggested that pulmonary disease in adults may be associated with chlamydiae. Tack *et al.* (1980) recovered *C. trachomatis* from the lower respiratory tract of 6 patients with pulmonary infections which varied from acute bronchitis to severe pneumonia. The latter appeared in 4 immunosuppressed patients from 3 of whom cytomegalovirus was also recovered. Three of the patients improved promptly after treatment with doxycycline or erythromycin, but two patients died. Immunofluorescence serology was performed on 4 patients, of whom 3 were immunosuppressed; no antibodies against *C. trachomatis* were found.

This report suggests the possibility that *C. trachomatis* is among the organisms which can colonize the respiratory tract in special circumstances, but the source of the infection and the pathogenesis of the clinical disease are unknown.

9

Lymphogranuloma venereum

Lymphogranuloma venereum (LGV) is a sexually transmitted disease caused by *C. trachomatis* serotypes L1, L2 and L3, which are distinguished from other strains by the micro-IF test (Wang and Grayston, 1970). These strains differ from oculo-genital strains not only antigenically but biologically; for example, they are more pathogenic for mice, and grow well in cell culture without centrifugation. Clinically, LGV differs from the syndromes caused by oculo-genital strains, for while these infect columnar epithelium, LGV organisms invade lymphatic tissue, and most of the effects of the disease are due to this. Whether the three LGV serotypes differ in pathogenicity is not known.

Epidemiology

The disease is of world-wide distribution, but it is particularly common in tropical and subtropical countries. Although its prevalence appears to be declining, many cases are still seen in the West Indies, East and West Africa, India, South-East Asia and South America. It is endemic in some areas of the United States. In the UK, LGV is uncommon, and infections have almost always been acquired overseas.

In sexually active populations in areas of high prevalence of LGV asymptomatic infections appear to be quite common, particularly in women. Among male homosexuals, symptomless rectal infections are also important. There have been suggestions that there may be an appreciable incidence of undiagnosed LGV in the UK (King, 1964). This idea arose through the discovery of high CF titres, and positive intradermal tests in patients attending STD clinics. It is quite possible that these positive results were due not to infection by LGV organisms but by the closely related oculogenital strains; these are common causes of infection in STD clinic populations, and the two infections cannot be differentiated by CF or intradermal tests.

Clinical manifestations

Primary genital lesion

The incubation period of LGV is difficult to assess because of the transitory nature of the initial lesion; it is believed to be between two and five days, although longer periods have been described. In men, the primary lesion may be on the penis, often in the coronal sulcus or, in the case of homosexuals, in the anorectum. In women, the fourchette is said to be the commonest site (Greenblatt, Dienst and Baldwin, 1959), but primary lesions also occur on the labia or in the vagina or cervix. The lesion is transient and painless, and presents as a small papule, vesicle or ulcer; men occasionally develop endourethral lesions, which cause a scanty mucopurulent discharge. Extragenital sites such as the finger and mouth are sometimes affected.

The histology of the primary lesion shows no specific features. It heals rapidly. In many patients with undoubted LGV there is no history or clinical evidence of a primary lesion (Alergant, 1957), and it is much more usual for patients to present with the next stage of the disease, inguinal adenopathy.

Inguinal adenopathy

Lymphadenopathy usually appears between two and six months after the infecting coitus, but much longer intervals have been described. Inguinal adenitis is much commoner in men than in women. This may be because of the lymphatic drainage of the genital area. The penis and vulva drain into the inguinal lymph nodes, but the upper vagina and cervix into the external and internal iliac nodes; thus only women with primary lesions on the vulva would develop inguinal adenopathy.

In the majority of patients inguinal gland involvement is unilateral. A firm painful mass develops, which usually involves several groups of inguinal and even femoral nodes. Biopsy performed at this time shows small masses of epithelioid cells, with multinucleated giant cells scattered through the gland (Sheldon and Heyman, 1947). Spontaneous resolution of the infection may occur, but the formation of multilocular abscesses is more likely. Enlargement of nodes above and below the inguinal ligament constitute the 'sign of the groove', which is said to be diagnostic of LGV. After the development of suppuration, spontaneous rupture of one or more abscesses may occur: the contents vary from thin yellow fluid to purulent or caseous material. Healing is often slow, and in a small proportion of patients drainage of pus continues for months or even years. When the healing process predominates, contracted scars develop.

Involvement of deep iliac lymph modes may lead to a presumptive diagnosis of appendicitis (Law, 1943) or pelvic peritonitis. Axillary or submaxillary lymphadenopathy and abscess formation may follow primary LGV infection of the finger or mouth.

Constitutional symptoms

These are variable, and are not present in all patients; they are not necessarily related to the severity of the local disease (King, 1964), but are often present at the stage of lymph gland involvement or when suppuration is occurring. Fever, headache, anorexia, nausea, vomiting and myalgia are the commonest symptoms (Abrams 1968). White cell counts are usually normal, but the ESR may be raised.

Ano-rectal syndrome

This important manifestation of LGV comprises proctitis, rectal stricture and sometimes peri-rectal abscesses and the formation of fistulas. It is commoner in women than in men. Proctitis can occur very early in the course of LGV. In women, it is thought to result from extension of infection from the initial vulval or vaginal lesion to the rectum via the lymphatics of the recto-vaginal septum (King, 1964). In men, on the other hand, most cases of LGV proctitis are thought to follow anal coitus, during which direct infection of the rectal mucosa by LGV organisms has occurred.

In either event, a patient with LGV proctitis complains of bowel disturbances and the passage of blood, mucus and pus. Proctoscopy or sigmoidoscopy reveals that the mucous membrane of the anal canal and rectum is congested, granular and oedematous. Punctate haemorrhages may be present, and the epithelium bleeds easily and is covered by a mucopurulent exudate; superficial ulceration or polypoid masses may be seen as the infection progresses. Histology shows a non-specific granulomatous inflammatory process (Miles, 1959).

Proctitis without stricture is the earliest sign of ano-rectal LGV, and the prognosis of the disease if recognised and treated at this point is excellent. In the absence of treatment the proctitis continues, and the formation of fibrous tissue will in many patients lead to the development of rectal stricture after a few months to several years. The process of stricture formation may be complicated by perirectal abscess, fistula in ano and recto-vaginal fistula (Annamunthodo and Marryatt 1961). Stricture without proctitis is uncommon and seems to be confined to women. In these patients there is scarring of the rectal wall suggestive of earlier proctitis with recovery. It is doubtful whether rectal stricture occurs without antecedent proctitis (Miles, 1959).

Patients with rectal strictures due to LGV present with symptoms of chronic large bowel obstruction with or without symptoms of proctocolitis. Radiology shows changes suggestive of colitis as well as the presence of stricture. These are tubular or funnel shaped and of varying length; they usually begin 3–5 cm from the anal margin; multiple stricutres can occur (Annamunthodo and Marryatt 1961). In a few patients, obstructive symptoms from stricture may become so severe that abdominoperineal excision of the rectum and the establishment of a colostomy may be necessary.

The ano-rectal syndrome is an important complication of LGV whose treatment may present many problems. It has been suggested that LGV may sometimes predispose to malignant change in the ano-rectal area, and indeed in other areas such as the penis and vulva (Rainey, 1954; Pund and Lacy, 1951). Whether the development of carcinoma in patients with longstanding LGV is due to the effects of chronic inflammation, a specific response to infection with LGV agents, or simply coincidental is not known.

Elephantiasis of the genitalia

This occurs in both men and women; it seems to occur less often now than in the past. It has been attributed to both lymphatic obstruction and active chronic inflammation. Hypertrophic changes in the vulva occur, and there may be polypoid growths and chronic ulceration; in some patients, associated proctocolitis is present (King, 1964). Secondary necrotic changes may lead to much loss of tissue, hence the name 'esthiomene', literally 'eating away', which is sometimes given to the condition. Elephantiasis of the male genitalia due to LGV is rare, but undoubtedly occurs.

Other manifestations

Urethritis may be a late development in LGV; it has been described in association with the ano-rectal syndrome, and occurs in both men and women. The whole urethra may be involved, and strictures, fistulas and extensive urethral damage may follow.

Uncommon manifestations of LGV include meningitis, arthritis/tenosynovitis, cardiac involvement and pneumonia. Some patients show abnormalities of serum proteins; reversal of the albumen/globulin ratio may occur, particularly in chronic infections (Saad *et al.*, 1961). Immunoglobulins may be elevated, particularly those of IgA class (Lassus, Mustakiallio and Wagner, 1970; Schachter and Dawson 1978).

Differential diagnosis

Most cases of LGV occur in developing countries, where facilities for complex investigations may not be available. In these areas diagnosis may depend on clinical examination supplemented by simple laboratory aids. Furthermore, LGV may present with a variety of symptoms and lesions which may resemble, or even be associated with, other diseases. The diagnosis of LGV for these reasons may not be easy. Early LGV must be distinguished from other causes of genital ulceration and/or lymphadenopathy.

Syphilis

In its primary stage this disease also presents with genital ulceration and enlargement of regional lymph nodes. The primary chancre of syphilis is non-indurated and evanescent. The lymphadenopathy of syphilis is painless, and abscess formation does not normally occur; that of LGV is often painful, and abscess formation is common. Serological tests for syphilis are mandatory in any patient with genital ulceration with or without regional adenopathy, and should be repeated at least once after an interval of up to twelve weeks. Biological false positive reactions are not unusual in LGV so at least one, and preferably two, specific tests (e.g. TPHA and FTA-ABS) should be included.

Genital herpes

This disease is like LGV in presenting with genital ulceration and lympha-denopathy which is often painful. In genital herpes infections, however, ulceration is often multiple and painful, and it is slower to heal than the transient primary lesion of LGV; conversely, the duration of adenopathy is shorter in herpes infections than in LGV. Isolation of Herpes simplex virus from the vesicles or ulcers will confirm the diagnosis of genital herpes infection.

Chancroid

This disease is also common in tropical and subtropical areas, and both genital ulceration and suppurative adenitis occur. Chancroidal ulceration is usually multiple, acutely painful and slow to heal. The isolation of *Haemophilus ducreyi* from the ulcers or from pus from the abscesses will enable a firm diagnosis to be made.

Bacterial lymphadenitis

Infection of inguinal lymph nodes, which may progress to suppuration, may be caused by superficial infection of the tissues of the legs, feet, buttocks or the perianal area, and should certainly be sought in any patient with unexplained adenopathy. Specimens from infected areas, or pus from an inguinal abscess, may be cultured to identify the infecting organism; the identification of pyogenic bacteria does not necessarily exclude LGV, as the lymphadenopathy of this disease may become secondarily infected.

Other diseases

Cat scratch disease is a possible cause of suppurative inguinal adenitis. Its cause is unknown (at one time it was erroneously attributed to chlamydial infection). It is diagnosed by a history of contact with cats, finding a primary lesion (usually on the leg) and a positive intradermal test.

It is not likely that inguinal adenopathy due to LGV will often be confused with an **irreducible inguinal hernia**, although this error has occurred. A more common difficulty, particularly in areas where the prevalence of LGV is low, arises in the diagnosis of **inguinal adenopathy of unknown origin.** Such nodes are quite properly biopsied to exclude a reticulosis or other serious disease, but it is important, particularly in patients who have recently travelled overseas, that the possibility of LGV is borne in mind and appropriate diagnostic tests (*see* below) included in the investigations.

Diagnosis of the ano-rectal syndrome

The differential diagnosis of this syndrome is from other causes of proctitis and rectal stricture. Acute proctitis due to LGV in male homosexuals must be distinguished from other causes of proctitis in these patients (Kazal, Sohn and Corrasco, 1976). It is important to remember that rectal infections from oculogenital strains of *C. trachomatis* may be difficult to distinguish, both clinically and serologically, from LGV proctitis (*see* below).

Proctocolitis with or without stricture formation will require differentiation from other causes of inflammatory bowel disease, particularly ulcerative colitis and Crohn's disease. These patients are likely to present to the gastro-enterologist or rectal surgeon rather than to the genito-urinary physician, and their diagnosis will not be pursued further here.

Mixed infections

Double or multiple infections are commonplace among patients with sexually transmitted iseases, and it is not unusual for patients with LGV to have other infections (Alergant, 1957). In establishing the diagnosis of LGV, therefore, it is important to exclude the possibility of associated infections by appropriate laboratory tests. At least, serological tests for syphilis and cultures for *N. gonorrhoeae* should be performed, but these tests may need to be supplemented according to local conditions.

Laboratory diagnosis

The Frei test

Frei (1925) introduced a delayed hypersensitivity test for the diagnosis of LGV. The original antigen was heat-inactivated pus obtained from an inguinal abscess of a patient with the disease. Subsequently, antigens were prepared by growing the LGV agent in laboratory animals and, later, in yolk sacs. The last method was used for preparing the commercial Frei antigen, which is no longer obtainable.

The test is performed by intradermal inoculation of 0.1 ml of antigen and 0.1 ml of a control preparation. The test is read after 48 hours; a 5 mm indurated area at the test site, with no reaction at the control site, is regarded as a positive result.

The Frei test is not specific for LGV and will sometimes give positive reactions in other chlamydial diseases, e.g. oculo-genital infections and psittacosis. Moreover, like other delayed hypersensitivity tests such as the Mantoux test, the Frei test cannot distinguish between past and current infection; this may be a real problem in areas where LGV is prevalent. The test usually becomes positive within a few weeks of infection, and a positive reaction may persist for many years, even for life. Some patients with confirmed LGV have negative Frei tests (Schachter *et al.*, 1969). Because of its lack of sensitivity and specificity, the Frei test has been largely abandoned. Nevertheless, it should be stated that many physicians with a large clinical experience of LGV found it a useful diagnostic aid.

The complement fixation test

This test is widely used. It is group-specific, and either LGV or *C. psittaci* antigens, grown on yolk sac, are used. In LGV, the CF test becomes positive within a week or two of infection (Alergant, 1957). In untreated patients it may remain positive for life. After treatment, a fall in titre may occur, but in some patients the serology is unchanged.

Classical serology demands that for a CF test to be diagnostic, a rising titre of antibodies must be demonstrated. This is rarely practicable in LGV; many patients already have high titres when they first present, or they may be unable to attend for repeated tests. In practice, a single CF test is often the only serological test which is possible. Patients with active LGV commonly have titres of 64 or more (Schachter and Dawson, 1978). It must be remembered that the LGV CFT is a group-reactive test, and that cross reactions with other chlamydial diseases such as oculo-genital infections may occur. However, the titres of antibodies in these infections is rarely more than 16. Thus although a demonstration of high titres in the LGV CF test is not conclusive proof of current LGV infection, it is undoubtedly a useful diagnostic aid; it should be considered with other clinical and laboratory findings.

Micro-immunofluorescence test

The micro-IF test (page 30) is sensitive, and allows specific identification of oculo-genital strains of *C. trachomatis* to be made. LGV strains are broadly reactive in this test, so that patients with the disease have high micro-IF titres against all ocular and oculo-genital strains (Wang and Grayston 1974). Thus this test is of no more diagnostic value for LGV than the LGV CFT.

Isolation of LGV agent

This provides a definitive diagnosis. Specimens from any infected site may be examined, aspirated pus being the best material. Microscopy is of no value, but inoculation of fertilized hens' eggs was successfully used for many years. Cell culture systems (Chapter 3) are preferable if they are available.

Histopathology

Histological studies on LGV indicate that the basic lesion is one of proliferation of large mononuclear cells to form aggregates; later, central necrosis with a PMN reaction, leading to the formation of stellate abscesses, is seen. The picture has been described in detail by Sheldon and Heyman (1947).

Some workers believe that the histology of LGV is sufficiently distinctive to allow a reasonably accurate diagnosis, and recommend biopsy as an adjunct to other diagnostic procedures.

Comment

With the exception of isolation of the agent, none of the above laboratory investigations will provide a definitive diagnosis of LGV. Precision in diagnosis requires a careful consideration of the history and clinical manifestations combined with the best use of the laboratory services which are available. In LGV we see the paradox that the most sophisticated laboratory procedures are available in developed countries, where the incidence of LGV is low. It is to be hoped that good laboratory facilities for diagnosis will soon be available in developing countries, for there are many questions about LGV which need answering. The epidemiology, and the role of symptomless carriers, require more study. The pathogenicity of the three known serotypes has not been decided. The relationship between LGV and neoplasms should be studied further. Above all, perhaps, the possibility of simplified diagnostic methods and improvements in treatment should be investigated.

10

Treatment

Chlamydial infections are persistent. Mammalian species, including man, infected by *C. psittaci* may shed infective organisms for years. LGV is essentially a chronic infection, and its effects may persist for a prolonged period. Trachoma is likewise a chronic disease which may remain active, or liable to recurrences, almost indefinitely. Infections with genital chlamydiae show a similar behaviour. Although adult and neonatal inclusion conjunctivitis have been regarded as self-limiting infections, in both conditions active disease persists in some patients for a long time (see page 39). In the genital tract there is good evidence that cervical infections persist for many months (McCormack *et al.*, 1979; Rees *et al.*, 1977a). In men, the results of placebo treatment of *Chlamydia*-positive NGU, and the demonstration of continuing chlamydial infection after the treatment of gonorrhoea, both show that the organisms can remain viable in the urethra for several weeks, and probably for much longer (Prentice, Taylor-Robinson and Csonka, 1976; Johannisson, Sernryd and Lycke, 1979; Vaughan-Jackson *et al.*, 1977). Babies with untreated chlamydial pneumonia shed organisms for at least two months (Beem and Saxon, 1977).

Since spontaneous cure is unlikely, genital infections by *C. trachomatis* require active treatment. Even mild or asymptomatic infections may lead to major complications, and a high level of chlamydial infection in a community inevitably means a correspondingly high level of potentially serious disease in men, women and infants. This level is directly related to the vigour with which efforts are made to contain it by the diagnosis and effective treatment of infected people.

Choice of drug

This depends in the first place on activity against *C. trachomatis in vitro* (*see* Chapter 2). In the laboratory, the most active drugs are, 1. the tetracyclines, including the newer derivatives minocycline and doxycycline; 2. the macrolides erythromycin and rosaramicin; 3. rifampicin and its derivatives. Sulphonamides show less activity, and the penicillins are ineffective. Although rifampicin is very active against *C. trachomatis in vitro*, resistance can be easily induced in the laboratory (Ridgway, Boulding and Lam Po Tang, 1980). Furthermore, some authorities believe that this drug should be restricted to the treatment of tuberculosis, so it seems unlikely that rifampicin will find a place in the therapy of chlamydial infection, but some of its analogues may prove to be of value. The majority of clinical trials have been devoted to tetracyclines and the macrolides. The sulphonamides have also been studied, although to a lesser extent.

The second kind of choice is between a drug which is selectively concentrated in genital tissue such as the prostate and one which is not. Although theoretically such concentration might be thought desirable, it is not clear whether this point is of clinical importance. Among the tetracyclines, minocycline and doxycycline are concentrated in the prostate, and both erythromycin and rosaramicin also give good penetration.

It is desirable that an antichlamydial drug should also be active against other genital tract pathogens. A familiar example of this is the problem of treating synchronous gonococcal and chlamydial infections, which will be discussed below. In the treatment of *Chlamydia*-positive NGU the use of a broad spectrum antibiotic has advantages; both rifampicin and sulphonamides have given poor clinical results, even though *C. trachomatis* is not re-islated. This may be due to lack of activity against other associated bacteria, in particular *U. urealyticum*, and in this respect the broader activity of the tetracyclines is probably an advantage.

Finally, it is important that the drug regimen selected should be simple, free from side effects and (if possible) inexpensive. In STD clinics generations of physicians have become accustomed to single-dose therapy for gonorrhoea, but it is unlikely that single-dose therapy for chlamydial infections will be possible (certainly not with existing antimicrobial agents), desirable though this may be.

In clinical practice, the antimicrobial drugs most often used for the treatment of chlamydial infections are the tetracyclines (oxytetracycline, tetracycline hydrochloride, minocycline and doxycycline), and erythromycin compounds; of the latter, erythromycin estolate is hepatotoxic and should not be prescribed, so most physicians prescribe either erythromycin base or erythromycin stearate.

Treatment of eye disease

A vast experience of treating these infections, particularly trachoma, has accumulated during the last 30 years, and we will summarize this only briefly. Schachter and Dawson (1978) may be consulted for a more detailed presentation.

Trachoma

Among the problems of management in this disease are some which are only too familiar to the genito-urinary physician — failure of compliance in therapy, the effects of secondary infection, and the pressure of re-infection through living conditions on the one hand and sexual promiscuity on the other. However, the major complications of trachoma caused by scarring — distortion of the upper tarsus, trichiasis and entropion — do not have a counterpart in the genital tract, and to this extent the treatment of genital chlamydial infections is simpler.

Prolonged topical tetracyclines or erythromycin are effective in trachoma, but topical sulphonamides are ineffective. Systemic tetracyclines give good results, but they cannot be given to children under the age of seven years (an important target group) or to expectant or nursing mothers. Sulphonamides are effective orally, particularly if combined with local tetracycline therapy, but their use is limited because of allergic reactions and the development of erythema multiforme. It is agreed that in hyperendemic areas it is desirable to treat the whole community.

The effect of therapy not only on *C. trachomatis* but on associated bacterial pathogens is important in deciding the outcome, and Jawetz (1969) has suggested that the success of tetracyclines is in part due to suppression of this bacterial superinfection. While acute infections may be cured by such therapy, the treatment of chronic chlamydial eye disease is far more difficult, so that high dosage and prolonged administration of tetracyclines is advisable. He believes that while these drugs do suppress the growth and replication of *C. trachomatis* they may fail to eliminate the microbe completely from an infected host. This opinion has often been quoted, and sometimes misinterpreted as an opinion that chlamydial infections are incurable. It should be noted that this is not what Jawetz said. His perfectly valid reflections on the natural history of trachoma and the effect of antibacterial drugs upon it should not be extrapolated and applied to the very different area of genital tract infections.

Inclusion conjunctivitis

Experience in treating this eye infection is relevant to chlamydial genital infections, since both are usually caused by the same serotypes of *C. trachomatis*. Treatment with systemic tetracyclines leads to rapid improvement of inclusion conjunctivitis (Dawson *et al.*, 1970). Conjunctival follicles may persist for several months before they disappear. Oral tetracycline 250 mg six hourly for three weeks has been recommended; courses of less than one week may be followed by recurrence.

For patients unable to take tetracyclines, erythromycin derivatives (*see* below) may be used in equivalent dosage. While oral sulphonamides have also been effective, they give an unacceptable number of side effects and their use is not now recommended. Topical therapy with tetracycline has only a limited effect on inclusion conjunctivitis, and systemic treatment is preferred: this is particularly advantageous in view of the common association of chlamydial genital tract infection with inclusion conjunctivitis.

Treatment of chlamydial genital infections in men

Treatment of NGU

Cell culture techniques have been used to study the effect of antimicrobial therapy on men with *Chlamydia*-positive NGU, endo-urethral specimens being collected before therapy and on one or more occasions after its completion.

Tetracyclines

It is clear from the data that tetracycline derivatives are highly effective against *C. trachomatis* infection of the urethra (Table 10.1). It is very unusual to re-isolate the organisms within two weeks of the completion of treatment, and early treatment failures, when they occur, are probably due to poor compliance. On longer follow up, urethral chlamydiae do occasionally reappear. Handsfield *et al.* (1976) obtained positive urethral cultures from a few patients more than six weeks after tetracycline therapy but thought that re-infection rather than relapse was responsible. We have followed patients for up to twelve weeks after therapy with oxytetracycline and have also occasionally re-isolated *C. trachomatis*, but usually when re-infection was either proved or probable (Oriel, Ridgway and Tchamouroff, 1977a). The difficulty of distinguishing between relapse and re-infection is a familiar problem in treatment trials in STD, which can be avoided only by selecting for study a confined group of men, eg the servicemen on an aircraft carrier in the classical investigation of Holmes, Johnson and Floyd (1967).

Table 10.1   Results of treatment of men with *Chlamydia*-positive NGU with tetracyclines

Authors	Drug and dosage	Re-examination		
		Duration of therapy	Time after completion of therapy	Number yielding chlamydiae/ number tested
Handsfield *et al.*, 1976	Tetracycline 500 mg 6 hourly	1 week	3 days	0/10
Oriel, Ridgway and Tchamouroff, (1977a)	Oxytetracycline 250 mg 6 hourly	2 weeks	1–2 weeks	1/31
Oriel, Reeve and Nicol, 1975a	Minocycline 100 mg twice daily	3 weeks	immediate	0/33
Prentice, Taylor-Robinson and Csonka, (1976)	Minocycline 200 mg stat 100 mg twice daily	6 days	immediate	1/12
Johannisson, Sernryd and Lycke, (1979)	Doxycycline 200 mg stat 100 mg daily	6 days	1 week	1/57

It is also clear from the data that the dose and duration of therapy with various tetracyclines appears to have little effect on the microbiological outcome. For example, there is no apparent difference between the results obtained with minocycline 100 mg twice daily taken for three weeks and 50 mg twice daily for one week (Oriel *et al.*, 1975a; Oriel and Ridgway, unpublished), or between tetracycline 250 mg or 500 mg four times daily taken for one week (Bowie, Yu and Fawcett, 1980). It should be noted, however, that effective regimens must be of at least six to seven days duration; shorter periods of treatment in our experience, and in that of others (Schachter, personal communication) may be followed by early recurrence.

Other antimicrobial drugs

The results of therapy of *Chlamydia*-positive NGU with regimens of erythromycin, sulphonamides and rifampicin are shown in Table 10.2. On short-term follow up, re-isolation of *C. trachomatis* is rare. Some men treated with erythromycin stearate 500 mg twice daily for two weeks and followed for up to twelve weeks became culture-positive again after a few weeks, but this was unusual and was mostly associated with probable reinfection. Rosaramicin is active against *C. trachomatis in vitro*, but has not yet been fully evaluated clinically.

Clinical response to therapy

Although antimicrobial agents may be effective against *C. trachomatis*, their action on the associated symptoms and signs of urethritis is variable; tetracyclines give good results, whereas sulphonamides, despite their antichlamydial effect, have a disappointing clinical activity. The same phenomenon can be seen with rifampicin, which is highly active *in vitro* against *C. trachomatis*. Coufalik, Taylor-Robinson, Csonka (1979) treated men with NGU with either rifampicin 600 mg daily for six days or with minocycline 200 mg stat followed

Table 10.2   Results of treatment of men with *Chlamydia*-positive NGU with erythromycin preparations, trimethoprim/sulphamethoxazole and rifampicin

Authors	Drug and dosage		Re-examination	
		Duration of therapy	Time after completion of therapy	Number yielding chlamydiae/ number tested
Oriel, Ridgway and Tchamouroff, (1977a)	Erythromycin stearate 500 mg twice daily	2 weeks	1–2 weeks	0/31
Johannisson, Sernryd and Lycke, (1979)	Erythromycin 500 mg twice daily	10 days	1–4 weeks	5/23
Bowie, et al., (1977)	Sulfisoxazole 500 mg 6 hourly	10 days	3–8 days	0/22
Johannisson, Sernryd and Lycke (1979)	Sulphamoxole 1 g twice daily for 1 day then 0.5g twice daily	9 days	16 days	0/20
Johannisson, Sernryd and Lycke, (1979)	Trimethoprim 160 mg/ sulphamethoxazole 800 mg twice daily	10 days	2–3 weeks	2/20
Coufalik, Taylor-Robinson and Csonka, (1979)	Rifampicin 600 mg once daily	6 days	2–3 weeks	1/53

by 100 mg twice daily for six days. *C. trachomatis* was re-isolated from 1 (2 per cent) of 53 initially *Chlamydia*-positive patients after treatment with rifampicin, and from 1 (2.5 per cent) of 40 after treatment with minocycline. However, the proportion of patients whose urethritis resolved completely was smaller after treatment with rifampicin (37 per cent) than after treatment with minocycline (68 per cent). These incomplete recoveries are presumably due to lack of therapeutic action against associated micro-organisms, including *U. urealyticum*. Even the use of tetracyclines, which give the best clinical response, is followed by a persistent urethritis in 10–15 per cent of patients treated for *Chlamydia*-positive NGU although cultures for *C. trachomatis* are negative.

Recommended treatment

Successful treatment of chlamydial urethritis means the elimination of *C. trachomatis* and the disappearance of the symptoms and signs of infection — namely, dysuria, urethral discharge, urethral leucocytosis and pyuria. By these criteria, tetracyclines give good results. While laboratory studies will indicate the sensitivity of a micro-organism to antimicrobial agents, the dose and duration of therapy can be decided only through clinical trials. The results of treatment trials do not, in our opinion, indicate that high dosage and prolonged courses of treatment with tetracyclines are necessary. While it is obviously essential to adopt curative therapy, over treatment is pointless.

A three week course of therapy has been used in several studies, but the case for such a prolonged course of treatment, with its attendant problems of compliance, has not been made. At the other end of the scale, it is known that treatment for less than one week is liable to be followed by recurrence. Like others, we have used tetracycline or oxytetracycline 250 mg six hourly for two weeks as routine treatment for chlamydial infection of the lower genital tract with good results. A two week course carries the advantage of protecting the patient from re-infection while sexual partners are being traced and treated. The data indicate that shorter courses of treatment, provided they are of at least a week's duration, also give good results, but the dose schedule must be rigorously adhered to, and there is little room for compliance failure. For these reasons we prefer the longer course. It must not be forgotten that tetracyclines chelate with heavy metal ions, so milk, milk products and antacids should be avoided during therapy.

The newer compounds minocycline and doxycycline are effective, and have the advantages of a simple twice or once daily dose schedule and perhaps greater penetration into urogenital tissues; they have the disadvantage of side effects, vestibular with minocycline, and gastro-intestinal with doxycycline. Again, high dosage is not necessary, and good results are obtained with minocycline 100 mg twice daily for two weeks, or doxycycline 200 mg stat followed by 100 mg daily for two weeks. Patients who are intolerant of tetracyclines should be given erythromycin; erythromycin base 250 mg six hourly, or erythromycin stearate 500 mg twice daily, may be given for two weeks. Sulphonamides, although they have activity against *C. trachomatis*, give such poor results in the treatment of NGU that they are no longer used.

After treatment, men with NGU need at least two follow-up examinations at intervals of one to two weeks. Culture for *C. trachomatis* should, of course, be negative. Patients with residual urethritis need careful evaluation. This may be due simply to slow resolution of the inflammatory process as happens, for example, in some patients with inclusion conjunctivitis; in others, associated infections are responsible, and a search must be made for *T. vaginalis*, Herpes simplex virus and other possible causes. If there is no apparent cause for persistent *Chlamydia*-negative urethritis in these circumstances, some physicians treat the patients empirically with a different antibiotic — e.g. erythromycin if tetracycline has been used before — but the value of this has not been established by controlled clinical trials.

Management of sexual contacts
The identification and treatment of infected sexual contacts is a vital part of the management of STD, and is essential for chlamydial infections. Failure in this respect can lead only to an increase in the prevalence of infection, and is no doubt a major reason for the escalating incidence of NGU which is seen in the UK and other countries at present. We recover *C. trachomatis* from the cervix of 60 per cent of female contacts of men with *Chlamydia*-positive NGU, and from the urethra of nearly 50 per cent of current male contacts of women with chlamydial cervical infections, and have no doubt that these infected people should receive treatment.

Contacts of patients with chlamydial infection should preferably not be treated unseen, but be interviewed and examined by a physician; some have associated infections which need treatment, and even if none of these is present compliance is improved if the necessity for treatment is explained personally. If facilities for the culture of *C. trachomatis* are available, only those patients who yield isolates need be treated. If there are no facilities, it is preferable for all contacts to receive appropriate treatment with an anti-chlamydial drug once associated infections have been excluded. Examination and treatment of contacts should be expeditious, to avoid the possibility of re-infection of the index cases.

Summary
A recommended schedule of treatment for *Chlamydia*-positive NGU is summarized in Table 10.3. (This therapy is also effective in most patients with *Chlamydia*-negative NGU.)

Table 10.3 Recommended routine management of NGU

---

1   Tetracycline/oxytetracycline 250 mg six hourly for two weeks
2   No milk, milk products or antacids during antibiotic therapy
3   No intercourse for three weeks after beginning therapy (condom if abstinence impossible)
4   Alcohol restricted during therapy
5   Examination of sex partners; epidemiological treatment after associated infections excluded
6   Follow-up examinations two and four weeks after beginning therapy

---

Treatment of epididymitis

Information on the treatment of other chlamydial infections in men is scanty. Therapy with tetracyclines is effective for men with *C. trachomatis* epididymitis (Berger *et al.*, 1978). The testicular swelling is often slow to resolve, and penetration into the inflamed tissue may be poor; for these reasons many physicians prolong treatment for two to three weeks. It is, of course, essential to examine and treat female sexual contacts of these men.

Treatment of chlamydial genital infections in women

Lower genital tract infection

Several studies on the effect of antimicrobial therapy on chlamydial infection of the cervix have been performed. Follow up has usually been for a relatively short time, but some long term follow up has been possible. Most investigations have concerned tetracycline, but erythromycin has also been used (Table 10.4).

Table 10.4 Results of treating women with cervical infection by *C. trachomatis* with tetracycline and erythromycin preparations

Authors	Drug and dosage	Duration of therapy (weeks)	Re-examination	
			Time after completion of therapy	Number yielding chlamydiae/ number tested
Oriel *et al.*, (1975a)	Minocycline 100 mg twice daily	3	immediate	0/24
Rees *et al.*, (1977a)	Oxytetracycline 250 mg 6 hourly	3	3–6 months	3/37
Waugh and Nayyar, (1977)	Triple tetracycline* one tablet twice daily	3	1 week	0/10
		1	3 weeks	0/44
Oriel and Ridgway, (1980)	Oxytetracycline 250 mg 6 hourly	2	1–2	2/70
	Erythromycin stearate 500 mg twice daily	2	1–2 weeks	0/70

*Tabs Deteclo (Lederle)

As with chlamydial infections in men, treatment with antichlamydial agents appears to be microbiologically successful. In the short term it is very unusual to re-isolate chlamydiae after such therapy, and the available data do not indicate that late recurrence occurs sufficiently often to be of importance. Thus in one of our own studies (Table 10.5) we found that in the majority of cases where *C. trachomatis* was re-isolated after oxytetracycline therapy it was likely that re-infection from an untreated sex partner rather than relapse was responsible — indeed in some cases it was possible to prove this by isolating the organism from the male urethra. The same point has been made

Table 10.5 Re-isolation of chlamydiae from women with cervical infections by *C. trachomatis* after treatment with oxytetracycline 250 mg six hourly for two weeks

Weeks after completion of therapy	Number yielding chlamydiae/ Number tested
1–2	2(1)/70
3–4	2(1)/38
5–6	1(1)/22
7–8	0/16
9–10	0/9

Figures in parenthesis indicate number of probable re-infections

by Tait *et al.* (1980), who treated a group of women with cervical chlamydial infection with a three week course of oxytetracycline 250 mg six hourly. Thirty-eight women were followed for between two and fourteen months, but *C. trachomatis* was re-isolated from only 5 women, and in 4 of these there was a strong possibility of re-infection.

The effect of therapy on the clinical signs of chlamydial infection of the cervix, like the signs themselves, are not well documented. However, Rees *et al.* (1977a) reported that in a group of 38 infected women exhibiting hypertrophic erosion who were followed for longer than four weeks after therapy the erosion became and remained simple; there was a corresponding reversion of mucopurulent cervical exudate to a nonpurulent secretion in the majority of patients.

If the examination of sexual contacts of men with chlamydial genital infection is desirable, it is no less so for contacts of infected women. This procedure is often omitted, but it is important, as nearly 50 per cent of current male partners of women with cervical chlamydial infection have a similar infection of the urethra.

Salpingitis

Therapy directed against a specific causal agent is used for salpingitis associated with *N. gonorrhoeae*, but with this exception treatment of salpingitis has been largely empirical (Thompson and Hager, 1977). Clinically, penicillin/ ampicillin and tetracycline are equally effective in the treatment of both gonococcal and non-gonococcal salpingitis, although there is a higher incidence of pelvic abscess after treatment of the latter (Cunningham *et al.*, 1977). There are no data specifically related to the effect of therapy on tubal *C. trachomatis* infection, but such data will certainly be needed if a major role for the organism in this disease is established. It would be desirable for microbiologically controlled studies to be performed to evaluate various regimens in both short and long term. Until then, treatment of women with salpingitis associated with *C. trachomatis* with full dosage of tetracyclines seems logical; it must not be forgotten that some women with gonococcal salpingitis have an associated chlamydial infection, and this must be borne in mind when planning therapy. Finally, the investigation of sexual contacts of women with salpingitis, although often overlooked, is clearly essential.

Recommended treatment

For **lower genital tract infections**, the same regimens of treatment which are effective for urethral chlamydial infections in men are effective for women. Tetracycline/oxytetracycline 250 mg six hourly for two weeks have given good results when used by many investigators. During pregnancy and lactation, erythromycin base 250 mg six hourly or erythromycin stearate 500 mg twice daily for two weeks should be substituted.

For **salpingitis** associated with *C. trachomatis* it is customary to use higher dosage, e.g. tetracycline/oxytetracycline 500 mg six hourly for two weeks, or equivalent dosage of erythromycin derivatives. Many physicians advise the addition of metronidazole 400 mg twice daily, as there is often an associated anaerobic infection.

Management of associated gonococcal and chlamydial infections

Men

The management of simultaneous infections of the urethra with *N. gonorrhoeae* and *C. trachomatis* will depend on whether culture facilities for *Chlamydia* are available. If they are, the initial penicillin/ampicillin/spectinomycin treatment for gonorrhoea will be followed, in patients yielding chlamydial isolates, by a full course of a tetracycline. If isolation facilities are not available, the physician has a choice. He can follow routine treatment for gonorrhoea and wait and see whether the patient develops PGU; if he does, he would normally be given a course of tetracycline, and if this is adequate *C. trachomatis*, if present, will be eliminated. Alternatively, the physician may decide to adopt antichlamydial treatment routinely, either by following immediate single-dose therapy for gonorrhoea with a course of tetracycline, or by using a tetracycline to treat gonorrhoea (e.g. tetracycline 500mg six hourly for one week), which will also cure an associated chlamydial infection. Neither of these choices is ideal, but single-dose therapy which cures both infections is not possible with existing antimicrobial agents; therefore the clinician perforce will have to adopt one of the measures outlined above.

Women

The association of chlamydial infection with gonorrhoea is commoner in women than in men, and is a particularly difficult problem since women do not develop an identifiable syndrome corresponding to PGU in the male. In our view, unless facilities for *Chlamydia* culture are available, there is no feasible alternative to including a tetracycline, or erythromycin, in the routine treatment for gonorrhoea.

Treatment of neonatal infections

Neonatal inclusion conjunctivitis
Since chloramphenicol has only a moderate antichlamydial activity, local

chloramphenicol, which is commonly prescribed for conjunctivitis, is unsatisfactory for the treatment of neonatal inclusion conjunctivitis. Tetracycline eye ointment, applied four hourly for two to three weeks, is commonly recommended for therapy (Rees *et al.*, 1977c). The success of this treatment is questionable. Although these workers report that re-isolation of *C. trachomatis* is unusual after therapy, Schachter and Dawson (1978) refer to a failure rate of close to 50 per cent, and we ourselves have repeatedly re-isolated the organism after this treatment. Many failures may be due to inadequate application of the ointment, but both poor penetration and re-infection are also possible.

Because of the unsatisfactory results of topical treatment it is better if neonatal chlamydial eye infection is treated with systemic erythromycin as well as topical tetracycline for three weeks (Ridgway and Oriel, 1977b). We have had no treatment failure with over fifty babies treated in this way.

The desirability of systemic treatment for neonatal inclusion conjunctivitis is strengthened by the observation that topical ocular therapy does not prevent respiratory tract colonization (Beem and Saxon, 1977); these workers reported that 10 of 11 babies with conjunctival infection persisting after local therapy yielded chlamydiae from the nasopharynx. Systemic treatment of chlamydial eye infections in these babies would be expected to reduce the possibility of pneumonia.

Pneumonia
Beem, Saxon and Tipple (1979) managed 11 patients with neonatal chlamydial pneumonia without specific antimicrobial therapy for between 10–60 days; all continued to shed chlamydiae, and none showed clinical improvement. In contrast, the same group treated 32 infants with either sulfisoxazole 150 mg/kg/day or erythromycin ethyl succinate 40 mg/kg/day for approximately fourteen days. All the infants stopped shedding chlamydiae soon after treatment began, and all improved clinically, usually within seven days of starting therapy. In 3 infants (1 treated with sulfisoxazole and 2 with erythromycin) *C. trachomatis* was re-isolated after the completion of therapy, but without recrudescence of clinical disease. The authors conclude that specific antichlamydial therapy is beneficial to infants with a confirmed chlamydial pneumonia syndrome, and might be justified on clinical grounds in infants who satisfy the diagnostic criteria if diagnostic facilities for *Chlamydia* are not available.

Prophylaxis
The application of one per cent silver nitrate drops at birth for the prevention of gonococcal ophthalmia neonatorum was introduced by Credé in 1880; it was very successful, and to this day is used in many countries, although no longer in the UK. Ocular prophylaxis with silver nitrate does not prevent chlamydial ophthalmia (Schachter *et al.*, 1979c). Because of this, and because in some populations chlamydial eye infections excede gonococcal infections by a factor of more than ten to one, the possibility of specific ocular prophylaxis with an antichlamydial agent has been considered.

Hammerschlag *et al.*, (1980) used erythromycin eye ointment for this purpose in a group of 24 babies born to women with confirmed chlamydial genital infection. None of the infants developed chlamydial conjunctivitis, but in 5 *C. trachomatis* was subsequently isolated from the nasopharynx. It seems likely that this kind of ocular prophylaxis may be effective against eye infections, but will not prevent the potentially more serious respiratory tract infections.

In communities with a high level of neonatal chlamydial infection the possibility of screening for cervical infections during pregnancy must clearly be considered. In the mean time, the mothers of babies with chlamydial infections must be investigated and treated; it is often more difficult to locate and treat the fathers or current male partners of these women, but it is clearly no less important.

Treatment of lymphogranuloma venereum

The natural history of LGV is variable, and spontaneous healing may occur; for these reasons controlled treatment trials are desirable, and it is a pity that it has been possible to conduct so few of these. There is general agreement that treatment early in the disease has the best chance of success. In chronic infections the presence of fibrosis and other structural changes reduces the benefit obtained from medical treatment, and surgery may be essential.

Sulphonamides

These were the first antimicrobial agents to be used for the treatment of LGV, and they are still favoured by some workers. In the early studies sulphathiazole or sulphadiazine were given orally in a dosage of 2–6 g daily for 5–14 days. Alergant (1957) gave sulphathiazole 1 g 6 hourly for 10–14 days, repeating the course if necessary after 1–2 weeks. Alternatively, sulfisoxazole (sulphafurazole) may be used, with a loading dose of 4 g followed by 500 mg 6 hourly for 21 days (Schachter and Dawson, 1978). The relative merits of different sulphonamide regimens have not been determined, but it is probable that provided full dosage is administered for 2–3 weeks the choice of sulphonamide is not critical. An advantage of these drugs is that they do not mask incubating syphilis.

Tetracyclines

These drugs have been used for the treatment of LGV since the late 1940s and there is no doubt about their efficacy. As with other chlamydial diseases, the optimal dose and duration of tetracycline therapy for LGV has not been decided; dosages of 1–2 g of tetracycline or oxytetracycline for 10 days–3 weeks have been recommended by different authors (King, 1964). A recommended standard course of therapy is tetracycline 250 mg 6 hourly for 3 weeks (Schachter and Dawson, 1978), but this regimen may have to be repeated if the clinical response is poor.

Different LGV strains may vary in their sensitivity to sulphonamides (Hurst *et al.*, 1950), but it is not clear whether this is important in clinical practice, as some workers have reported no difference in the therapeutic response of patients with LGV to sulphonamides or tetracyclines (Alergant, 1957; Greaves *et al.*, 1957). Although the tetracyclines are now widely used for therapy, it may be that the stage of the disease when treatment is begun is the most important predictor of success.

Other drugs

Penicillin and streptomycin are ineffective for LGV (Coutts, 1950). Chloramphenicol is relatively ineffective and may produce serious side-effects. Erythromycin, with its in-vitro activity against *C. trachomatis*, should be effective, but the drug has not been extensively evaluated against LGV. Rifampicin is highly active against chlaymdiae *in vitro*, and in one study has been shown to be clinically effective in the therapy of LGV (Menke, Schuller and Stolz, 1979).

Surgical measures

Inguinal abscesses should be aspirated, if necessary repeatedly, with a wide-bore needle; incision should be avoided. Some patients with inguinal adenopathy are very slow to respond to treatment, but this should still be by repeated courses of antimicrobial agents with aspiration when necessary; excision of the infected gland mass is not usually successful.

Patients with chronic rectal disease due to neglected LGV may respond to antibacterial drugs alone, but usually surgery is necessary. Miles (1957) has discussed the surgical procedures available, and these will not be reviewed here; surgery is in all cases preceded by an adequate course of chemotherapy. The surgical treatment of other late complications of LGV has been reviewed by King (1964).

General measures

Many patients with longstanding LGV are in poor general health through the effects of the disease, associated disorders and malnutrition; correction of co-existing diseases and dietary deficiences will be necessary. Patients with ano-rectal disease may be severely anaemic and need the administration of iron or blood transfusion. Even in those patients with LGV who are less seriously ill the provision of rest and adequate diet are helpful in the management of a disease which is often depressing and exhausting to the patient.

11

Discussion

During the last seventy years there have been periodic waves of interest in human chlamydial infections, each wave having been set in motion by a particular technical advance. If we are on the crest of such a wave now it is for two main reasons. First, there is a realization that in modern society sexually transmitted diseases and their associated disorders are common, important and a proper subject for study and research. Second, it is now plain that infections caused by *C. trachomatis* are among the most important of these, and in the introduction of cell culture and micro-immunofluorescence serology has provided the essential technology for their study.

In this chapter we attempt to draw together the threads of argument from the previous sections and to present some general statements about infection with genital strains of *C. trachomatis*.

Pathogenicity of *C. trachomatis*

Eye infections

The pathogenicity of *C. trachomatis* in the human eye is unquestioned. It was shown many years ago that isolates of the agent from patients with trachoma could reproduce the disease in man (Collier, Duke-Elder, and Jones, 1958). Similarly, experimental inoculation of chlamydiae derived from a baby with inclusion conjunctivitis into the eyes of an adult volunteer was followed by acute chlamydial eye disease (Jones, 1964). Koch's postulates have thus been satisfied for both ocular and genital strains of *C. trachomatis*.

The reality of attempting to separate the ocular diseases caused by these strains has been questioned, particularly by the group headed by Professor Barrie Jones at the Institute of Ophthalmology in London. It is pointed out that infection by genital serotypes may lead to an eye disease indistinguishable from trachoma (Jones, 1964); conversely, infection by ocular strains may result in inclusion conjunctivitis or superficial punctate keratitis rather than pannus or conjunctival scarring (Grayston and Wang, 1975). It is now usually accepted that a continuous spectrum of chlamydial eye disease exists, and that it is an over-simplification to make a rigid attribution of particular ocular syndromes to specific serotypes. Epidemiologically, however, hyperendemic trachoma on the one hand and paratrachoma on the other occur in vastly different settings. The matter is still undecided, but the clinical manifestations of chlamydial eye disease may to some extent depend on the severity of secondary bacterial infection and on the effects of re-infection by *C. trachomatis*.

In trachomatous communities, associated bacterial infections greatly influence the pathogenesis of the eye disease, perhaps by inducing more intense conjunctival or corneal inflammation with subsequent scar formation and pannus. A comparable process has been demonstrated in cats infected by the feline conjunctivitis agent, which belongs to the species *C. psittaci*; combined inoculation of *Streptococcus* spp. and this chlamydial agent led to a far more severe keratoconjunctivitis than the inoculation of either microbe alone (Darougar *et al.*, 1977).

Neonates whose eyes are infected by *C. trachomatis* may have concurrent bacterial infection, not only by *N. gonorrhoeae* but sometimes by other organisms. Rees *et al.* (1977c) relate early onset of the disease to these associated infections but it is not clear whether they aggravate the inflammation, although this would seem likely.

The pathogenicity of *C. trachomatis* in the eye may also be affected by immunological factors. Grayston and Wang (1975) have argued that chronic trachoma with its characteristic signs of pannus and conjunctival scarring occurs after re-infection and/or relapse and depends on immune reactions to the organism. A process of this kind might explain the pathogenesis of typical trachoma in non-endemic areas, the immunological background in these cases being the result of genital tract infection and reinfection by *C. trachomatis*.

Urethritis

While there is no doubt that *C. trachomatis* is a pathogen in the conjunctival mucosa, there has been some controversy over its role in urethritis in men. There is agreement that chlamydiae are an important cause of PGU; the organisms are consistently recovered from the urethra of men with PGU, but not from control groups without PGU (see page 48). *C. trachomatis* is not the only cause of PGU, but there is general agreement that it causes the majority of cases.

The situation with NGU may be less straightforward. *C. trachomatis* can undoubtedly cause NGU when it infects a previously normal urethra for the first time; in this group clinical evidence of infection is accompanied by isolation of the organism, seroconversion, and initially high titres of IgM antibody (Bowie, *et al.*, 1977). Is a similar primary causal role established for the majority of men with *Chlamydia*-positive NGU? The contrary argument has been skilfully deployed by Richmond, Hilton and Clarke (1972) and Richmond and Sparling (1976). It is derived from the following observations: 1. the failure to define an incubation period in *Chlamydia*-positive (or negative) NGU; 2. the increased isolation rate with increased duration of symptoms in men with NGU; 3. similar isolation rates in NGU and gonorrhoea, particularly when patients are matched for duration of symptoms; 4. the isolation of chlamydiae from some men with NGU who give no history of recent sexual exposure; 5, the presence of antibody in most men with *Chlamydia*-positive NGU even if their symptoms have lasted for only a few days.

To explain these observations, Richmond and her co-workers have suggested that chlamydial infections may persist in a latent form but can be reactivated by certain stimuli. Among these stimuli could be included (a) *N. gonorrhoeae* (resulting in high isolation rates in gonorrhoea and the induction of PGU), and (b) an unknown agent, the real cause of NGU. Thus the chlamydial isolation rate in NGU would increase with the duration of symptomatic urethritis induced by this unknown agent, and persistent latent chlamydial infections would account for the discrepant serological findings.

These arguments are perceptive, but in some respects may be too elaborate. Chlamydial infections may be severe or mild, and host responses may be such that only asymptomatic or subclinical disease results; this is true of all chlamydial infections. Furthermore, experience with ocular chlamydial disease suggests that with the passage of time chlamydiae become more difficult to isolate. We find no difficulty in accepting that the inflammatory insult of gonorrhoea may make it easier to recover *C. trachomatis* from patients with latent or subclinical infections. Although the data in fact indicate that the rate of recovery of chlamydiae from men with gonorrhoea is usually lower than from men with NGU, this does not vitiate the truth of the underlying concept.

It does not, however, seem necessary to introduce the operation of an unknown agent to explain the common association of *C. trachomatis* and NGU. None of the other microbes suggested as possible causes of NGU are significantly associated with *Chlamydia*, and it is difficult to argue about the significance of an entirely hypothetical agent. Nevertheless, there is no reason why one or more of the other microbes which cause NGU may not act jointly with *C. trachomatis* in pathogenesis, in the same way as urethritis may be due to the simultaneous operation of *N. gonorrhoeae* and *C. trachomatis*.

In summary, therefore, it seems likely that exposed populations, such as men attending STD clinics, will contain men with NGU in the following categories: 1. men experiencing their first attack of chlamydial urethritis, which may be clinically obvious or subclinical; some will have associated infections with other organisms, e.g. *U. urealyticum*. 2. men with a past history of urethritis who similarly have infections with *C. trachomatis* with or without other organisms. 3. men with NGU caused by non-chlamydial agents.

In clinical practice NGU is a disease of some complexity, but the facts that *C. trachomatis* is not the only cause, that mixed infections by chlamydiae and other microbes occur, and that mild and asymptomatic chlamydial urethral infections are quite common do not, in our view, imply that *C. trachomatis* is not pathogenic to the male urethra. Although inoculation of the human urethra with the organism has never been performed, all the evidence indicates pathogenicity.

Epididymitis

The studies of Berger *et al.* (1978) in Seattle strongly indicate that, at least in that area, *C. trachomatis* is a common cause of acute epididymitis in young men.

Whether in other areas chlamydial infection is the commonest cause of non-gonococcal epididymitis cannot be decided until more data are available, but it seems a reasonable assumption that in localities where chlamydial infection of the urethra is common much epididymitis will have a similar pathogenesis.

Acute epididymitis is undoubtedly a possible complication of NGU, particularly if procedures such as prostatic massage or urethral instrumentation are undertaken in untreated patients. How common the disease is as a complication of chlamydial NGU is not known; to determine this would require a prospective study of untreated men with chlamydial urethritis which would not be acceptable. But whether it is a common or a rare event, the fact that *C. trachomatis* is potentially pathogenic to the epididymis strengthens the necessity for adequate treatment of these urethral infections.

Cervical infection

It has proved difficult to define the effects of chlamydial infection of the cervix. In part, this is because many cervices from which *C. trachomatis* is recovered are completely normal, or show only cervical erosion, which is not an indicator of cervical disease. In part also, the terminology is inexact, and the word 'cervicitis' which is commonly used to describe cervical infection lacks clear definition. Finally, the cervix is a complex area subject to traumatic, infective and hormonal influences, which may make it difficult to interpret changes associated with the presence of one micro-organism. We have argued (page 59) that to equate urethritis in men with cervicitis in women may be dangerously misleading, and to this we would add a plea that the meaningless term 'non-specific genital infection' is now abandoned.

It is plain that cervical infection by *C. trachomatis* shows a wide spectrum of disease; this is also true for infection by *N. gonorrhoeae*. At one extreme, about half of women infected with chlamydiae have clinically normal cervices, or exhibit only cervical erosion. Among the remainder there are some who have pre-existing cervical disease unrelated to *Chlamydia*, but most show to a varying extent the changes of cervicitis, i.e. congestion, oedema and a purulent exudate. There is no doubt that many of these changes are the direct result of chlamydial infection, for they have been seen to develop in women studied prospectively who have been exposed to infection and to disappear, together with demonstrable chlamydiae, after antimicrobial therapy. However, it should be emphasized that none of these changes is specific to infection by *C. trachomatis*; they may be seen in women with other infections, or indeed in women infected simultaneously by chlamydiae and other micro-organisms. The cervical microfollicles visible by colposcopy in many women infected by *C. trachomatis* may be specific to this organism (page 58), but this has not yet been confirmed by controlled studies.

In exposed female populations there is much chlamydial cervical infection; for example about 20 per cent of women attending STD clinics in the UK are infected. In many women, host responses occasion a clinically silent condition. The very high isolation rates reported in gonorrhoea (up to 60 per cent in some series) may well be due in part to the reactivation of some of these quiescent chlamydial infections. There is no doubt that *C. trachomatis* can persist in infected cervices, certainly for many months and possibly for years. Whether in the long term these infection can cause either gynaecological disorders, in particular early abortion, fetal loss, premature labour or cervical dysplasia is not clear at present, but prospective and sero-epidemiological studies should provide answers to these questions.

Salpingitis

The part played by *C. trachomatis* in the pathogenesis of pelvic inflammatory disease has been much discussed recently. Early observations had suggested that the two might be related, and laparoscopy has now made it possible to recover chlamydiae directly from inflamed fallopian tubes (Mårdh *et al.*, 1977). These Swedish workers believe that in a high proportion of their patients with salpingitis the disease is caused by *C. trachomatis*. This is clearly a most important observation. Acute salpingitis, with its sequels of chronic PID, infertility and ectopic gestation, is a disease of major medical and economic importance. If *C. trachomatis* is a common cause of salpingitis, measures for the diagnosis, treatment and control of lower genital tract infection by the organism are of the utmost importance — at least as important as for *N. gonorrhoeae*, and perhaps more so since chlamydial infection is commoner. In addition, recommended treatment schedules for salpingitis would need modification to allow for the role of chlamydiae.

Data derived from the investigation of patients with salpingitis and from animal experiments have been described above (page 61) and certainly indicate that *C. trachomatis* can cause tubal inflammation. The crucial questions are, in which geographical areas, and how often? In Sweden, *C. trachomatis* appears to be the commonest cause of acute salpingitis; in that country the incidence of salpingitis has been increasing and that of gonococcal infections diminishing (Treharne *et al.*, 1979). The risk of acquiring acute salpingitis following chlamydial infection of the cervix is not known with certainty, but may be at least as high as occurs with *N. gonorrhoeae*.

The observations have not yet been repeated in other countries, and until they are we advocate caution. It would be unwise to assume that *C. trachomatis* is a major cause of salpingitis throughout the world. Its aetiology may well vary from country to country; in the USA for example, recent data (page 64) have not shown an association between chlamydial infection and salpingitis. This is not to deny the importance of the matter — indeed, it is too important for hasty judgements to be made. The potential role of *C. trachomatis* in PID requires careful evaluation in those countries, including the UK, where laboratory facilities are available and where chlamydial infection of the lower genital tract is known to be common. The meticulous studies of the Swedish group indicate the metholology which could usefully be employed.

Neonatal infections

Over seventy years ago it was known that *C. trachomatis* was pathogenic to the eye in neonates. Subsequent experience has shown that, like all chlamydial infections, neonatal inclusion conjunctivitis can be mild or severe, and result in clinical or subclinical disease. While these phenomena are familiar, neonatal respiratory infection by *C. trachomatis* has been identified only within the last few years. The pathogenesis of chlamydial pneumonia is not yet clear. It follows colonization of the upper respiratory tract by chlamydiae derived from a maternal genital infection; it is seen by most investigators as a direct pathogenic effect of the organisms on the lung, although in some of the published cases the possibility of a mixed infection, e.g. with cytomegalovirus, cannot be excluded. While Koch's postulates can obviously not be fulfilled in humans, a closely similar disease has been induced in primates by experimental inoculation of the respiratory tract with human genital chlamydiae (see page 21). In some communities there is no doubt from the results of prospective studies that there is a definable risk not only of inclusion conjunctivitis but of pneumonia in babies of mothers who are harbouring chlamydiae.

In contrast with neonatal inclusion conjunctivitis, which is common in many Western countries, nearly all the cases of chlamydial pneumonia which have been described have been in the USA. Whether paediatricians in other countries are failing to diagnose the pneumonia syndrome, or it is taking a different clinical form, or even is not occurring at all, cannot be decided at present. It would clearly be unwise to prejudge the issue; studies to determine the incidence of chlamydial pneumonia should be performed, particularly in those countries where chlamydial genital infection is known to be common.

The recovery of chlamydiae from several anatomical sites in neonates and the identification of resulting disease of the eye, the lung, and possibly the middle ear, has posed some interesting questions. By analogy with other chlamydial infections, might there be a subclinical form of the pneumonia syndrome which escapes diagnosis and treatment? If so, what is the long-term prognosis, and might it affect respiratory function in older children? Infection of the gastro-intestinal tract by strains of *C. psittaci* often causes disease in animals. *C. trachomatis* is less invasive, but it infects columnar epithelial cells in many areas, and has been recovered from the rectum in neonates. Is there infection of other parts of the gastro-intestinal tract, and do any of these cause clinical disease in infancy, or later?

Whether any of these speculations will be confirmed remains to be seen. However, the pathogenicity of *C. trachomatis* to at least some columnar epithelia in neonates is undeniable and has important consequences.

Influence of host responses

It has been argued that among the factors which aggravate the clinical course of trachoma are not only secondary bacterial infection but also re-infection of the eye by *C. trachomatis*. Successive chlamydial infections may thus lead to more severe disease through the operation of immune processes; as Wang and Grayston (1975) express it, 'trachoma is a disease of immunopathology'. There is a *C. psittaci* animal model which shows the same phenomenon, for successive inoculations of the eyes of guinea-pigs with the guinea-pig inclusion conjunctivitis agent leads to increasingly severe conjunctivitis (Darougar *et al.*, 1977).

The effect of secondary bacterial infection on genital infection by *C. trachomatis* can probably be seen in some cases of NGU, cervicitis and salpingitis. Do immune reactions due to previous chlamydial infection also modify the disease process? We see no evidence of this in NGU, and suggestions that successive chlamydial infections of the urethra might lead to urethral stricture formation appear to be unsubstantiated. Similarly, chlamydial disease of the lower genital tract in women does not appear to be immunologically mediated. However, in salpingitis hypersensitivity reactions are possible. It has been shown that in organ culture of human fallopian tubes tissue *C. trachomatis* is only weakly pathogenic to cells, and has no effect on ciliary function (see page 63). In the intact host, if *C. trachomatis* causes salpingitis, it is conceivable that immune reactions are involved. (There are those who believe that the pathogenesis of *Chlamydia*-associated salpingitis involves mixed infections.)

Another example of an immunological process may be furnished by neonatal chlamydial pneumonia. In this disease, the long incubation period and eosinophilia may indicate the development of hypersensitivity rather than a primary infection; Beem and Saxon themselves (1977) believed that this might be possible.

In infections with genital chlamydiae, therefore, we may see a mixture of pathological processes. Some conditions are the result of direct infection with *C. trachomatis*: for example, adult and neonatal inclusion conjunctivitis, some cases of NGU and most cases of PGU. In other chlamydial diseases — salpingitis, cervicitis, and probably some cases of NGU — the effects of secondary bacterial infection are seen, while in others the disease is conditioned by previous exposure to *C. trachomatis* — examples of this may be some cases of salpingitis and neonatal pneumonia. These considerations in no way indicate that genital strains of *C. trachomatis* are not pathogenic, but the way which their pathogenicity is expressed appears to be complex.

Epidemiology

The development of sensitive and specific micro-IF tests has made possible serological studies of population groups to discover the extent of their exposure to chlamydial infection. The antigens used in these tests have varied. Some workers have employed a broadly reactive LGV strain or a genital serotype as sole antigen, while others have used an array of individual or pooled genital and ocular serotypes (see page 31). Based as they are on single determinations of IgG antibody, these sero-epidemiological studies cannot indicate the extent of *current* chlamydial infection; for this, isolation procedures are needed. But serology does indicate the extent to which a group has been exposed to infection, and the more refined techniques can be used to show whether this infection was with ocular or genital strains of *C. trachomatis*, and to identify predominant serotypes.

Several serological studies have been published (Richmond and Caul, 1975; Wang *et al.*, 1977; Schachter and Dawson, 1978). About 25 per cent of sexually active men show detectable antichlamydial antibodies, and antibodies are present in 60 per cent of men attending STD clinics. Sexually active women show reactor rates of 50–70 per cent and prostitutes of 80 per cent. About 10 per cent of children under the age of fifteen are sero-reactive. Not surprisingly, among adults the antibodies are predominantly to genital serotypes.

There is a lack of knowledge about the development and duration of antibodies to *C. trachomatis*, but these surveys show evidence of a considerable exposure to chlamydial infection, at least among sexually active groups. The greater prevalence of antibodies in women in comparison with men might be explained as being the result of a longer duration of infection, or infection of a larger anatomical area, providing a greater immunological stimulus. An association between seropositivity and increasing sexual experience has been demonstrated by McComb *et al.* (1979) in a study of female college students, when it was found that the presence of antichlamydial antibodies bore a direct relationship to the lifetime number of sex partners. It is interesting that this study shows that some women with no sexual experience at all have serum antibodies against *C. trachomatis*. This is consistent with observations that approximately 10 per cent of children in some populations have significant micro-IF titres (Alexander *et al.*, 1977; Schachter and Dawson, 1978). The reason for this is not known. It has been conjectured that it is due simply to persistence of antibodies following a neonatal chlamydial infection, but the possibility of the continued presence of infecting organisms cannot be excluded.

There are some aspects of this sero-epidemiological work which are difficult to understand, and will not become clearer until the kinetics of immunological reactions to *C. trachomatis* are better understood. It is plain, though, that a major limitation of single IgG antibody measurements is their inability to distinguish current from past infection. For public health and control purposes it is obviously important to know the prevalence of current infection by *C. trachomatis* but there are practical difficulties in attempting to isolate the organism on a large scale, and few population groups have been studied in this way. The available data (*see* Tables 5.2, 6.1) indicate that chlamydial genital infection is present in a small proportion of symptomless sexually active men attending STD clinics. Such infections appear to be commoner in women, and it is probably as true for chlamydial infection as for gonococcal infection that the reservoir of asymptomatic infection is predominantly composed of women.

The results of sero-epidemiology and of cell culture are consistent with a view of *C. trachomatis* as a sexually transmitted organism, but direct evidence of venereal spread may be obtained only by investigating sex partners of individuals who are known to be infected. Several studies of this kind have been performed over the years (*see* Table 6.2); there is, for example, a striking difference between the cervical isolation rates of women whose male partners have *Chlamydia*-positive as opposed to *Chlamydia*-negative NGU. It is important in contact-tracing studies to distinguish between source contacts (individuals who, from the history, appear to have transmitted the disease) and secondary contacts (individuals who have been exposed to infection). This distinction is sometimes said to be impossible but, although the status of a contact may at times be uncertain, a reasonable assessment can often be made.

We have investigated source and secondary contacts of men with both *Chlamydia*-positive and *Chlamydia*-negative NGU, and the results are summarized in Table 11.1. They give good evidence for the infectivity of *C. trachomatis*. The higher levels of infectivity shown by source in comparison with secondary contacts of men with *Chlamydia*-positive NGU are not seen in contacts of men with *Chlamydia*-negative NGU. The 12–14 per cent isolation

Table 11.1 Isolation of *C. trachomatis* from female contacts of men with NGU

Name of disease	Type of contact	Number examined	Number yielding *C. trachomatis*	Percentage positive
Chlamydia-positive NGU	source	36	30	83
	secondary	51	23	45
Chlamydia-negative NGU	source	44	6	14
	secondary	34	4	12

rate in these latter women appears to be the background for the group, as we see similar isolation rates in unselected women whose contact history is unknown.

In these studies the index cases have been male, but women with chlamydial infection diagnosed on routine examination can be used as index cases for the investigation of infectivity in the opposite direction. We have examined male contacts of these women, and found that about half yielded *C. trachomatis* from the urethra (these men were usually symptomless, and showed a very low clinical level of urethritis).

These contact tracing techniques can also be applied to women with gonorrhoea. Like others, we have found that about 40 per cent of these women yield *C. trachomatis* from the cervix. In our studies we have also found that while chlamydial isolates are obtained from 47 per cent of women who are secondary contacts of men with *Chlamydia*-positive gonorrhoea, they are also obtained from 32 per cent of women who are secondary contacts of men with *Chlamydia*-negative gonorrhoea. These results strongly suggest that some women with gonorrhoea had a cervical chlamydial infection before they were infected by the gonococcus. Whether these infections were latent and reactivated by *N. gonorrhoeae*, or whether they were simply subclinical, cannot be determined from these data.

Latency

A latent infection with *Chlamydia* is, by definition, present if the organisms are alive, but not replicating; in subclinical infections, on the other hand, the organisms are replicating but the clinical response to infection is small. There has been much discussion about latency, but this has not been supported by good clinical evidence. In the laboratory it has been possible to establish latent infection in strains of *C. psittaci* through nutritional depletion of the media and through multiple passage of infected cells (Hatch, 1975; Officer and Brown, 1961). It is possible that a temporary latency of *C. trachomatis* may follow incubation in the presence of antimicrobial agents under some conditions (see page 17). Clinical evidence of the existence of latency is meagre. Inclusions have been found in conjunctival scrapings without the presence of clinical eye disease (Hanna *et al.*, 1968), but sensitive cell culture techniques for the detection of replicating organisms were not available when this work was performed.

Clinically inapparent infections are commoner with all kinds of chlamydial disease; they are seen in human psittacosis and in various animal infections with *C. psittaci*, in LGV, in chlamydial eye disease and in genital tract infections. Whether latent infections in the true sense of the term also occur has not been proved, attractive though latency may be as a concept to explain some epidemiological findings.

Conclusions

The epidemiology of genital chlamydial infection is complex. There can be no doubt that *C. trachomatis* is sexually transmissible. Although not as infectious as *N. gonorrhoeae* (Lycke *et al.*, 1980), there is still a substantial risk of infection in those who are exposed to it. Such exposure is usually through heterosexual intercourse, and much less often through anal intercourse between homosexual men. Oro-genital contact has not been established as a regular route of infection.

Some men with *Chlamydia*-positive NGU are experiencing a primary infection. Others are having subsequent re-infections, and in a few a chronic urethritis is present which, because it is not severe, has escaped diagnosis and treatment. All these men are infectious to others.

Much chlamydial infection in women is clinically silent and persists as a chronic symptomless infection for months or years. These conditions remain potentially infectious until they are treated or die out. In addition, there is a probable 50 per cent chance of a woman with genital infection by *C. trachomatis* transmitting the organisms to her babies' eyes, causing inclusion conjunctivitis; about half of the infants with eye infections will develop pneumonia or other systemic chlamydial disease, and others may develop systemic infections without antecedent eye disease. In both men and women chlamydial infection may spread from initially infected sites to cause complications, of which the most serious are epididymitis and salpingitis.

What is the outcome of untreated genital infection? Little is known of this, and it is unlikely that prospective studies will be possible because of the risk of complications in untreated patients (Paavonen *et al.*, 1980). It may be assumed that some infections eventually resolve through the operation of host defences; conceivably, some become latent and then persist indefinitely.

The majority of chlamydial infections (but not all) excite a serological response. IgG antibodies will then persist for periods of time which will depend on the intensity and duration of infection, and probably on host factors. Whether these antibodies are protective seems unlikely. It has been suggested that following infection a temporary immunity may develop (Taylor-Robinson and Thomas, 1980); if this occurs it must be short lived, because we have often documented re-infection soon after therapy in both men and women. Some animal models, particularly guinea-pig inclusion conjunctivitis, seem to show a resistance phenomenon (Murray, 1977), but care must be taken in extrapolating experience with *C. psittaci* into the very different world of human *C. trachomatis* infections.

Some patients with gonorrhoea have an associated infection by *C. trachomatis*. In some, the infections have probably been transmitted from a source contact simultaneously. This cannot account for all these double infections, and there can be no doubt that some patients (particularly women) had chlamydial infection before exposure to *N. gonorrhoeae*; whether these infections were subclinical, or whether they were latent and reactivated by the gonococcus, is not known. These patients seem to us to be the best group in which to study the feasibility of latent human chlamydial infections. Latency, if it exists, is an important phenomenon, for it would obviously influence the success of conventional control measures.

From the beginning of clinical and laboratory investigation of chlamydial genital infection it has been clear that this is intertwined with ocular infections by these organisms. This is seen in neonatal inclusion conjunctivitis, and adult inclusion conjunctivitis in Western societies is inevitably associated with genital infection by the same organism in the patient, the patient's sexual contacts, or both.

Is laboratory diagnosis necessary?

The techniques for the laboratory diagnosis of oculogenital chlamydial infection have been discussed in Chapter 3, and their sensitivity compared in Table 3.1. The diversity of these procedures, and the controversies which surround some of them, are bewildering to those who are contemplating a laboratory service for the identification of *C. trachomatis* infections. The choice of methods will depend on the level of diagnostic service required and on the laboratory resources which are available.

Direct microscopy of specimens stained by Giemsa or indirect fluorescent antibody staining has the attraction of simplicity, but rigorous technical control is necessary, and the method is too insensitive for the diagnosis of genital infections. For the diagnosis of inclusion conjunctivitis, however, microscopy is valuable; Giemsa staining is satisfactory in neonatal disease, and FA for both neonatal and adult varieties.

The diagnostic value of serology is particularly difficult to evaluate, as directly contradictory views have been expressed by workers in this field. We are unconvinced that serology, for either local or systemic antibodies, is at present sufficiently reliable to be used as an alternative to culture for the diagnosis of urethritis, cervicitis or salpingitis. Serology is often useful for the diagnosis of LGV and for other systemic chlamydial diseases such as neonatal pneumonia, but even in these conditions attempts should be made to isolate the organism from suitable specimens, if possible.

There has been much discussion, especially in the UK, on whether a diagnostic service for *C. trachomatis* should be available, particularly to STD clinics where it is presumed that the majority of genital chlamydial infections present. Are culture techniques sufficiently cost effective to justify such a service, and should this be selective or, like culture for *N. gonorrhoeae* and syphilis serology, be available for all patients? This matter has been discussed in several recent publications (Richmond *et al.*, 1980; Taylor-Robinson and Munday, 1980; Willcox *et al.*, 1979; Richmond and Oriel, 1978). It has not been proposed that a diagnostic service is unnecessary, but some have suggested that a consideration of the natural history of genital chlamydial infection indicates ways in which the demands could be much reduced.

It is argued that treatment of NGU with an adequate course of a tetracycline or of erythromycin normally cures both *Chlamydia*-positive and *Chlamydia*-negative NGU clinically, and eliminates chlamydiae, if present, from the urethra. *C. trachomatis* is uniformly sensitive to tetracyclines, and erythromycin-resistant strains are very rare. Therefore it is concluded that investigation of men with NGU to ascertain whether or not their urethritis is chlamydial is unnecessary, and the disease can be managed quite satisfactorily along traditional lines. The problem of the association of *C. trachomatis* with *N. gonorrhoeae* could be solved if the routine treatment of gonorrhoea included an adequate course of a tetracycline or other antichlamydial agent (see Chapter 10). Again, chlamydial isolation attempts would be unnecessary.

A similar approach could be taken towards women. About one third of isolates of *C. trachomatis* from women attending STD clinics in the UK come from contacts of men with NGU. It is proposed that routine epidemiological treatment of all women in this category with a tetracycline or erythromycin would make it unnecessary to attempt to diagnose chlamydial infection. Over-treatment would not occur, since contacts of men with *Chlamydia*-negative NGU might also benefit from this therapy. Since a substantial number of women with gonorrhoea also have a chlamydial infection, a treatment regimen which includes a tetracycline, as advised for men, should be used (see page 95). The adoption of these procedures for female contacts of men with NGU and for women with gonorrhoea would result in the treatment, and presumed cure, of the great majority of chlamydial infections in women who attend STD clinics. There would be some women infected by *C. trachomatis*, perhaps about 10 per cent of the total, who do not fit into the above categories; the further suggestion is made that since some of these women have clinical cervicitis they could be treated on clinical grounds. Thus, except for children and a few special cases in adults, the need for a diagnostic service could be reduced to vanishing point.

These arguments are ingenious, but it must be realized that they are economic rather than scientific. It is a basic principle of microbiology that pathogenic organisms causing disease, or which may induce disease in others, should be identified, and *C. trachomatis* is such an organism. These proposals involve a loss of precision in diagnosis and the sacrifice of the principle 'diagnosis before treatment' which would never be countenanced for other infections. Blind therapy of infectious diseases with antimicrobial agents has been condemned for a quarter of a century, and it would be a pity if this were re-introduced, particularly into the confused area of so-called 'non-specific urethritis' and 'non-specific genital infection' at a time when diagnostic accuracy and rational therapy are at last beginning to be a possibility.

There are in addition some practical objections to dispensing with laboratory isolations. In some patients with subclinical disease the identification of chlamydiae may provide the only reason for antimicrobial treatment. Much contact tracing, particularly of secondary male contacts of infected women, cannot be attempted unless it is known that the women are infected. Re-isolation of *C. trachomatis* after treatment may occur, through failure in compliance or re-infection, and this will escape recognition in women unless culture facilities are available. Finally, the accurate diagnosis of infection in special groups such as babies will be facilitated if the laboratory procedures are controlled by the examination of heavily infected groups. Our own experience of having had available for the last four years a routine culture service for *C. trachomatis* leaves us with no doubt that this is an essential facility for a modern clinic dealing with sexually transmitted and related diseases.

We recognize that there are many practical difficulties in achieving this. There are problems in persuading the authorities to provide financial backing for the service, and laboratory space and technical staff are often scarce. For these reasons some limitations of the demands must be accepted until greater resources, or perhaps simpler diagnostic techniques, become available. Attention should be given to those groups known to be at risk for chlamydial infection yet who are unlikely to receive antichlamydial therapy. These will comprise men and women with gonorrhoea (unless tetracyclines are an integral part of their routine therapy), women with unknown contact histories attending STD clinics for routine investigation, babies with possible chlamydial infections and some adults with inflammatory eye disease. In gynaecological practice, a culture service for *C. trachomatis* would be of value for elucidating the cause of inflammatory cervical disease and salpingitis. We do not advocate routine culture of the urethral specimens in men with NGU in ordinary circumstances but it may be useful in some cases, particularly in men with borderline urethritis. Provided routine epidemiological treatment is given, culture of specimens from a sex partner of a man with NGU is not necessary if she is the only contact, but if she has other partners culture for chlamydiae should be performed to indicate the need for further contact tracing. Widespread screening of low-risk populations with cell culture is a waste of time and should not be undertaken.

It is therefore possible to envisage a limited diagnostic service. It is important to include a group known to be heavily infected by chlamydiae as a control; women with gonorrhoea fulfil this condition admirably. Economies could be made by centralizing some basic services. For example, tubes containing coverslip monolayers could be prepared in bulk in regional laboratories and supplied to local laboratories. It is, however, essential that incubation and examination of cultures is performed locally. This does not in itself present much difficulty for any microbiology laboratory with competence in routine culture procedures.

Control of genital chlamydial infection

The basic principles for the control of a sexually transmitted disease are familiar, and may be summarized:

1. Recognition by the medical authorities that the disease is important.
2. Provision of facilities for the diagnosis and treatment of the disease.
3. Identification of sex contacts and their examination to identify or exclude infection.
4. 'Epidemiological' treatment, i.e. full therapeutic doses of antimicrobials to individuals recently exposed to the infection, while awaiting the results of laboratory tests (the desirability of 'epidemiological' treatment

is disputed by some authorities, particularly in the UK).

5. Screening of high-risk groups; possibly screening in pregnancy for the prophylaxis of neonatal disease.
6. Training of medical and paramedical personnel in clinical and laboratory aspects of the disease.
7. Relevant health education for the general public.

When these principles are applied to genital chlamydial infection it is obvious that control is a long way off. Whether the infection is generally regarded as important is questionable; many medical authorities unfortunately still regard *C. trachomatis* as an esoteric subject for laboratory research but not of great clinical significance. Diagnostic services are not generally available in any country. In present circumstances it is futile to speak of control of chlamydial infection. As interest increases and the necessary technology becomes available it will no doubt become possible to devote the same efforts to the control of chlamydial genital infection as are currently given to the traditional infections, syphilis and gonorrhoea.

This is in the future, but there are several areas in which useful action can be taken immediately.

1. NGU must be properly treated with full courses of antimicrobials; many regimens in use in STD clinics are not adequate to cure chlamydial infection, although they may mitigate the symptoms.
2. Examination and epidemiological treatment of sex partners of men with NGU is mandatory.
3. Treatment regimens for gonorrhoea will need adjustment to take account of concomitant chlamydial infection.
4. Neonatal prophylaxis should be revised, particularly in high risk areas. Crédé's method of prophylaxis of neonatal eye infections will not eradicate *C. trachomatis*, but other methods may be effective. This is an urgent research priority.
5. Above all, perhaps, there should be provision of at least limited diagnostic facilities for *C. trachomatis* in all large deparments dealing with STD.

We are not pessimistic about the future. Admittedly, there are large gaps in knowledge. The basic processes of infection of cells by *C. trachomatis* are not well understood. The epidemiology of chlamydial genital infection is in some respects mysterious. Serological responses and their practical value in diagnosis are poorly understood. There is a lack of knowledge of the action of antimicrobial agents against chlamydiae. The long struggle to control the infection has not yet begun. Yet in the last two decades there have been enormous advances, and although in some ways resources are pitifully small recognition is now dawning that chlamydial genital infection is a danger to the health of many young men and young women and to the well-being of their children. From this recognition nothing but good will come.

Appendix

Laboratory procedures

Cytological techniques

Giemsa stain

Air dry smears of clinical material, or cover-slip cell cultures, then fix in methanol for ten minutes.

Replace methanol with freshly diluted Giemsa stain (Difco Laboratories, West Molesey, Surrey; dilute one part of stock concentrate with nine parts of phosphate buffer).

Stain for thirty minutes.

Rinse off Giemsa with phosphate buffer, and wash twice with buffer pH 6.8.

Allow smear to dry, mount and examine under oil immersion with bright field illumination.
Cover-slip cell cultures may also be examined using a ×40 objective and dark ground illumination.

Iodine stain

Air dry smears or cover-slip cell cultures, then fix in methanol for ten minutes.
Replace methanol with ten per cent Lugol's iodine, and stain for five minutes.
Run off iodine, and blot smear.
Allow to dry, mount and examine with a ×40 objective and bright field illumination.

Isolation techniques

I UDR-treated McCoy cells (after Reeve, Owen and Oriel, 1975).

Materials
McCoy cells   Growth medium: Eagle's minimal essential medium (MEM), supplemented with fetal calf serum (10% of V/V), glutamine (1% of ×100 concentrate containing 2 M glutamine), 7.5% bicarbonate (1.4%), vitamins (1% of Flow Laboratories ×100 concentrate, and gentamicin (1% of stock solution containing 1000 mg/1).

Transport medium: to 100 ml growth medium prepared as above, add: 1 ml glucose (3M stock solution), 1 ml amphotericin B (250 mg/l stock) and 1 ml vancomycin (1000 mg/l stock).

The medium is dispensed in 2 ml aliquots into tightly capped plastic tubes (7 ml bijoux).
Plastic tubes for culture: 10 ml tubes with flat bottom (Brunswick, High Wycombe), to take a 12 mm cover-slip (Solmedia Ltd, London E17).

Cover-slips should be washed and heat sterilized.

IUDR solution:
a) 5-iodo-2-deoxyuridine (Sigma Ltd, London), 1.25 mg/ml in dimethyl sulphoxide (10% V/V in distilled water). (Store at +4°C in darkness).
b) working concentration of IUDR is 25 mg/1 IUDR in growth medium.

Method
Treatment of cells   Seed McCoy cells in Nunc 81 cm² tissue culture flasks, at 3 × 10^6 in 15 ml of growth medium. Cells should be confluent after four days at 37°C. Remove growth medium, and wash cells in phosphate buffered saline. Add 2 ml of 0.25% trypsin; as soon as the cell sheet begins to fall off the flask, remove trypsin. Re-suspend cells in growth medium. Count, and dilute cells to give 10^5 cells per ml using growth medium plus 25 μg/ml IUDR.

One ml of this suspension is added to each 10 ml plastic tube containing a cover-slip. The tubes are incubated vertically at 37°C. Cells are ready for use after three to seven days.
Inoculation   Remove IUDR supplemented growth medium and replace with 1 ml of the transport medium containing the swab (squeeze swab against the side of the transport tube to express material). Centrifuge tubes for one hour at 3000 **g**, preferably at 35–37°C. Incubate tubes vertically for 48–72 hours at 37°C.
Examination of cultures   After incubation, remove medium and replace by methanol. Allow cells to fix for ten minutes. Cover-slip may now be stained with Giemsa or iodine, and examined as described above.

Cycloheximide treated McCoy cells (after Ripa and Mårdh, 1977)

Materials
As above, with cycloheximide (20 mg/l) substituted for the IUDR solution.

Method
Cells are initially prepared as above, and diluted to 2.5×10^5 McCoy cells/ml of growth medium in the 10 ml plastic tubes containing a cover-slip. Allow to incubate at 37°C for 24 hours, then remove medium.

Add one ml of specimen (prepared as above) plus 0.1 ml (20 mg/l) of cycloheximide (final concentration 2 mg/l). Centrifuge tubes at 3000 **g** for one hour. Incubate at 37°C for 72 hours, fix, stain and examine as above.

Serological technique
Whole inclusion immunofluorescence (after Richmond and Caul, 1975)

Material
Polytetrafluorethylene (PTFE) coated microscope slides (C. A. Hendley and Co., Loughton, Essex). Prepare slides by washing overnight in 5% MHCL. Rinse ×10 in tapwater, then ×5 in distilled water, followed by methanol and acetone. Sterilize in hot air oven at 160°C for a holding time of one hour.

Fluorescein conjugated anti-human gamma globulin (Wellcome MFO1, Fluorescent Antibodies anti-human globulin (sheep)). Incident or transmitted light fluorescence microscope.

Method
Preparation of slides   Seed tissue culture bottles (see above) with 3.5×10^6 McCoy cells, in 15 ml of growth medium plus (25 μg/ml of IUDR). Incubate at 37°C for three to five days.

Add 1 ml stock strain of *C. trachomatis* at a concentration of 10^6 inclusion forming units ml of growth medium, and incubate at 37°C for a further 48 hours.

Remove growth medium, wash with PBS buffered saline and add 2 ml of 0.25% trypsin. Re-suspend in growth medium, and centrifuge at 1000 G for 5 minutes. Re-suspend pellet in 5 ml of growth medium and disperse cells using a pasteur pipette.

Place one drop of the cell suspension on each well of the PTFE coated slides. Place slides in a moist box, add a small piece of solid CO_2 and seal. Incubate at 37°C for 8 hours.

Fix cells in acetone for 30 minutes. Check for presence and character of inclusions by staining one slide with Giemsa or iodine stain.

Slides may now be stored at −70°C until required.

Test proper
Dilute patient's serum, positive and negative control sera 1/10 for screening. Add one drop of diluted serum to each well on the slide, and incubate for one hour at 37°C.

Wash in phosphate buffered saline.

Add one drop of fluorescein labelled anti-IgG to each well, and incubate in a moist box for one hour at room temperature. Wash in phosphate buffered saline, mount in fluorescence mounting fluid, and examine by fluorescence microscopy.

Sera positive on screening should be further titrated against the positive and negative controls.

References

Abrams, A. J. (1968). Lymphogranuloma venereum. *Journal of the American Medical Association* **205,** 199–202.

Alani, M. D., Darougar, S., Burns, D. C. MacD., Thin, R. N. and Dunn, H. (1977). Isolation of *Chlamydia trachomatis* from the male urethra. *British Journal of Venereal Diseases* **53,** 88–92.

Alergant, C. D. (1957). Lymphogranuloma inguinale in the male in Liverpool, England, 1947 to 1954. *British Journal of Venereal Diseases* **33,** 47–51

Alexander, E. R., Chandler, J., Pheifer, T. A., Wang, S-P., English, M. and Holmes, K. K. (1977). Prospective study of perinatal *Chlamydia trachomatis* infection. *Nongonococcal urethritis and related infections,* p. 148–152 edited by Holmes, K. K. and Hobson, D., American Society for Microbiology, Washington DC.

Alexander, E. R., and Chiang, W. T. (1967). Infection of pregnant monkeys and their offspring with TRIC agent. *American Journal of Ophthalmology* **63,** 1145–1153.

Al-Hussaini, M. K., Jones, B. R. and Dunlop, E. M. C. (1964). Genital infection in association with TRIC virus infection of the eye, II Cytology. Preliminary report. *British Journal of Venereal Diseases* **40,** 25–32.

Annamunthodo, H. and Marryatt, J. (1961). Barium studies in intestinal lymphogranuloma venereum. *British Journal of Radiology* **34,** 53–57.

Armstrong, J. A. and Reed, S. E. (1967). Fine structure of L.G.V. agent and the effect of penicillin and 5 F–U. *Journal of General Microbiology* **46,** 435–444.

Arth, C., von Schmidt, B., Grossman, M. and Schachter, J. (1978). Chlamydial pneumonitis. *Journal of Pediatrics* **93,** 447–449.

Ashley, C. B., Richmond, S. J. and Caul, E. O. (1975). Identification of the elementary bodies of *C. trachomatis,* in the electron microscope, by an indirect immunoferritin technique. *Journal of Clinical Microbiology* **2,** 327–331.

Ballard, R. C., Block, C., Koornhof, H. J. and Haites, B. (1979). Delayed hypersensitivity to *Chlamydia trachomatis* — cause of chronic prostatitis? *Lancet* **II** 1305–1306.

117

Barron, A. L., White, J. W., Rank, R. G. and Soloff, B. L. (1979). Target tissues associated with genital infection of female guinea pigs by the chlamydial agent of guinea pig inclusion conjunctivitis. *Journal of Infectious Diseases*, **139**, 60–68.

Becker, Y. and Zackay-Rones, Z. (1969). Rifampicin — a new antitrachoma drug. *Nature* **222**, 851–853.

Bedson, S. P. and Bland, J. O. W. (1934). The developmental forms of the psittacosis virus. *British Journal of Experimental Pathology* **15**, 243–247.

Beem, M. O. and Saxon, E. M. (1977). Respiratory-tract colonisation and a distinctive pneumonia syndrome in infants infected with *Chlamydia trachomatis*. *New England Journal of Medicine* **296**, 306–310.

Beem, M. O., Saxon, E. and Tipple, M. A. (1979). Treatment of chlamydial pneumonia of infancy. *Pediatrics* **63**, 198–203.

Bell, S. D. and McComb, D. E. (1967). Differentiation of trachoma bedsoniae in vitro. *Proceedings of the Society for Experimental Biology and Medicine*. **124**, 34–39.

Berger, R. E., Alexander, E. R., Monda, G. D., Ansell, J., McCormick, G. and Holmes, K. K. (1978). *Chlamydia trachomatis* as a cause of acute "idiopathic" epididymitis. *New England Journal of Medicine* **298**, 301–304.

Bernkopf, H., Mashiah, P. and Becker, Y. (1962). Susceptibility of a Trachoma Agent Grown in FL cell cultures to antibiotics and a Sulfa drug. *Proceedings of the Society for Experimental Biology and Medicine* **111**, 61–67.

Blyth, W. and Taverne, J. (1974). Cultivation of TRIC agents: a comparison between the use of BHK 21 and irradiated McCoy cells. *Journal of Hygiene*, Cambridge **72**, 121–128.

Bowie, W. R., Alexander, E. R., Floyd, J. F., Holmes, J., Miller, Y. and Holmes, K. K. (1976). Differential response of chlamydial and *Ureaplasma*-associated urethritis to sulphafurazole (sulfasoxazole) and aminocyclitols, *Lancet* **II**,, 1276–1278.

Bowie, W. R., Alexander, E. R. and Holmes, K. K. (1977). Chlamydial pharyngitis? *Sexually Transmitted Diseases* **4**, 140–141.

Bowie, W. R., Alexander, E. R. and Holmes, K. K. (1978). Etiology of postgonococcal urethritis in homosexual and heterosexual men: roles of *Chlamydia trachomatis* and *Ureaplasma urealyticum. Sexually Transmitted Diseases* **5**, 151–154.

Bowie, W. R., Lee, C. K. and Alexander, E. R. (1978). Prediction of efficacy of antimicrobial agents in treatment of infections due to *C. trachomatis. Journal of Infectious Diseases* **138**, 655–659.

Bowie, W. R., Wang, S-P, Alexander, E. R., Floyd, J., Forsyth, P. S., Pollock, H. M., Lin, J. S. L., Buchanan, T. M. and Holmes, K. K. (1977). Etiology of nongonococcal urethritis: evidence for *Chlamydia trachomatis* and *Ureaplasma urealyticum. Journal of Clinical Investigation* **59**, 735–742.

Bowie, W. R., Yu, J. S. and Fawcett, A. (1980). Tetracycline for nongonococcal urethritis: two grams versus one gram for 7 days. *Current Chemotherapy and Infectious Diseases*, p. 1277. Edited by Nelson, J. D., Grassi, C. American Society for Microbiology, Washington DC.

Braley, A. E. (1938). Inclusion blennorrhea. A study of the pathogen changes in the conjunctiva and cervix. *American Journal of Ophthalmology* **21**, 1203–1208.

Braley, A. E. (1939). Relation between the virus of trachoma and the virus of inclusion blennorrhea. *Archives of Ophthalmology* **22**, 393–398.

Brewerton, D. A., Caffney, M., Nicholls, A., Walters, D., Oates, J. K. and James, D. L. O. (1973). Reiter's Disease and HLA–27. *Lancet* **II**, 996–998.

Burns, D. C. MacD., Darougar, S., Thin, R. N., Lothian, L. and Nicol, C. S. (1975). Isolation of *Chlamydia* from women attending a clinic for sexually transmitted diseases. *British Journal of Venereal Diseases* **51**, 314–318.

Byrne, G. I. and Moulder, J. W. (1978). Parasite-specified phagocytosis of *C. psittaci* and *C. trachomatis* by L an HeLa cells. *Infection and Immunity* **19**, 598–606.

Caldwell, H. D. and Kuo, C. C. (1977). Purification of a *Chlamydia trachomatis* specific antigen by immunoadsorption with monospecific antibody. *Journal of Immunity* **118**, 437–441.

Carr, M. C., Hanna, L. and Jawetz, E. (1979). Chlamydiae, cervicitis and abnormal Papanicolaou smears. *Obstetrics and Gynaecology* **53**, 27–30.

Collier, L. H., Duke-Elder, S. and Jones, B. R. (1958). Experimental trachoma produced by cultured virus. *British Journal of Ophthalmology* **42**, 705–720.

Collier, L. H. and Sowa, J. (1958). Isolation of trachoma virus in embryonate eggs. *Lancet* **1**, 993–996.

Coufalik, E. D., Taylor-Robinson, D. and Csonka, G. N. (1979). Treatment of nongonococcal urethritis with rifampicin as a means of defining the role of *Ureaplasma urealyticum*. *British Journal of Venereal Diseases* **55**, 36–43.

Coutts, W. E. (1950). Lymphogranuloma venereum: a general review. *Bulletin of the World Health Organisation* **2**, 545–562.

Cox, H. R. (1938). Use of yolk sac of developing chick embryo as medium for growing Rickettsiae of Rocky Mountain spotted fever and typhus groups. *Public Health Reports (Washington)* **53**, 2241–2247.

Croy, T. R., Kuo, C. C. and Wang, S. P. (1975). Comparative susceptibility of eleven mammalian cell lines to infection with trachoma organisms. *Journal of Clinical Microbiology* **1**, 434–439.

Cunningham, F. G., Hauth, J. C., Strong, J. D., Herbert, W. N. P., Gilstrap, L. C., Wilson, R. H. and Kappus, S. S. (1977). Evaluation of tetracyclines or penicillins and ampicillins for treatment of acute pelvic inflammatory disease. *New England Journal of Medicine* **296**, 1380–1383.

Darougar, S., Cubitt, S. and Jones, B. R. (1974). Effect of high speed centrifugation on the sensitivity of irradiated McCoy cell culture for the isolation of *Chlamydia*. *British Journal of Venereal Diseases* **50**, 308–312.

Darougar, S., Jones, B. R., Kinnison, J. R., Vaughan-Jackson, J. D. and Dunlop, E. M. C. (1972). Chlamydial infection. Advances in the diagnostic isolation of *Chlamydia*, including TRIC agent from the eye, genital tract and rectum. *British Journal of Venereal Diseases* **48**, 416–420.

Darougar, S., Kinnison, J. R. and Jones, B. R. (1971). Chlamydial isolates from the rectum in association with chlamydial infection of the eye or genital tract. 1. Laboratory aspects. Trachoma and Related Disorders. *Excerpta Medica, Amsterdam*, Edited by Nichols, R. L. pp. 501–506.

Darougar, S., Monnickendam, M. A., El-Sheikh, H., Treharne, J. D., Woodland, R. M. and Jones, B. R. (1977). Animal models for the study of chlamydial infections of the eye and genital tract. In *Non-gonococcal Urethritis and Related Infections*, p. 186. Edited by Hobson, D. and Holmes, K. K. American Society for Microbiology, Washington DC.

Darougar, S., Treharne, J. D., Minassian, D., El-Sheikh, H., Dines, R. J. and Jones, B. R. (1978). Rapid serological test for diagnosis of chlamydial ocular infection. *British Journal of Ophthalmology* **62**, 503–508.

Davies, J. A., Rees, E., Hobson, D. and Karayiannis, P. (1978). Isolation of *C. trachomatis* from Bartholin's ducts. *British Journal of Venereal Diseases* **54**, 409–413.

Dawson, C. R. and Schachter, J. (1967). TRIC agent infections of the eye and genital tract. *American Journal of Ophthalmology* **63**, 1288–1298.

Dawson, C. R., Schachter, J., Ostler, H. B., Gilbert, R. M., Smith, D. E. and Engleman, E. P. (1970). Inclusion conjunctivitis and Reiter's syndrome in married couples. *Archives of Ophthalmology*, **83**, 300–306.

Digiacomo, R. F., Gale, J. L., Wang, S-P. and Kiviat, M. D. (1975). Chlamydial infection of the male baboon urethra. *British Journal of Venereal Diseases* **51**, 310–313.

Dunlop, E. M. C. (1975). In *Recent Advances in Sexually Transmitted Diseases* Edited by Morton, R. S. and Harris, J. R. W., p. 290, Churchill Livingstone, London.

Dunlop, E. M. C., Darougar, S., Hare, M. J., Treharne, J. D. and Dwyer, R. St.C. (1972). Isolation of *Chlamydia* from the urethra of a woman. *British Medical Journal* **1**, 386.

Dunlop, E. M. C., Freedman, A., Garland, J. A., Harper, I. A., Jones, B. R., Race, J. W., du Toit, M. S. and Treharne, J. D., (1967). Infection by Bedsoniae and the possibility of spurious isolation: 2. Genital infection, disease of the eye, Reiter's disease. *American Journal of Ophthalmology* **63**, 1073–1081.

Dunlop, E. M. C., Hare, M. J., Darougar, S. and Jones, B. R. (1971a) Chlamydial infection of the urethra in men presenting because of "non-specific" urethritis. In: Trachoma and Related Disorders. Edited by Nichols, R. L.. *Excerpta Medica, Amsterdam* 494–500.

Dunlop, E. M. C., Hare, M. J., Darougar, S. and Jones, B. R. (1971b) Chlamydial isolates from the rectum in association with chlamydial infection of the eye or genital tract: II clinical aspects. In: *Trachoma and Related Disorders* pp. 507–512. Edited by Nichols, R. L. Excerpta Medica, Amsterdam.

Dunlop, E. M. C., Hare, M. J., Darougar, S., Jones, B. R. and Rice, N. S. C. (1969). Detection of Chlamydia in certain infections in man. II Clinical Study of Genital Tract, Eye, Rectum and Other Sites of Recovery of Chlamydia. *Journal of Infectious Diseases* **120**, 463–472.

Dunlop, E. M. C., Harper, I. A., Al-Hussaini, M. K., Garland, J. A., Treharne, J. D., Wright, D. J. M. and Jones, B. R. (1966). Relation of TRIC agent to "non-specific" genital infection. *British Journal of Venereal Diseases* **42**, 77–87.

Dunlop, E. M. C., Jones, B. R. and Al-Hussaini, M. K. (1964). Genital infection in association with TRIC virus infection of the eye. III. Clinical and other findings. Preliminary report. *British Journal of Venereal Diseases* **40**, 33–42.

Dunlop, E. M. C., Vaughan-Jackson, J. D., Darougar, S. (1972). Chlamydial infection. Improved methods of collection of material for culture from the urogenital tract and rectum. *British Journal of Venereal Diseases* **48**, 421–424.

Dunlop, E. M. C., Vaughan-Jackson, J. D., Darougar, S., and Jones, B. R. (1972b). Chlamydial infection: incidence in "non-specific" urethritis. *British Journal of Venereal Diseases* **48**, 425–428.

Dwyer, R. St. J., Treharne, J. D., Jones, B. R., Herring, J. (1972). Results of micro-immunofluorescence tests for the detection of type-specific antibody in certain chlamydial infections. *British Journal of Venereal Diseases* **48**, 452–459.

Embil, J. A., Ozere, R. L. and MacDonald, S. W. (1978). *Chlamydia trachomatis* and pneumonia in infants: report of two cases. *Canadian Medical Association Journal* **119**, 1199–1203.

Eschenbach, D. A., Buchanan, T. M., Pollock, H. M., Forsyth, P. S., Alexander, E. R., Lin, J-S., Wang, S-P., Wentworth, B. B., McCormack, W. M. and Holmes, K. K. Polymicrobial etiology of acute pelvic inflammatory disease. *New England Journal of Medicine* **293**, 166–171.

Evans, R. T. and Taylor-Robinson, D. (1979). Comparison of various McCoy cell treatment procedures used for detection of *C. trachomatis*. *Journal of Clinical Microbiology* **10**, 198–201.

Falk, H. C. (1946). Interpretation of the pathogenesis of pelvic infection as determined by cornual resection. *American Journal of Obstetrics and Gynecology* **52**, 66–73.

Fehr, (1900). Endemische bad Konjunktivitis. *Berliner Klinische Wochenschrift* **37**, 10–11.

Ford, D. K. (1968). Non-gonococcal urethritis and Reiter's Syndrome. *Canadian Medical Association Journal* **99**, 900–910.

Freedman, A., Al-Hussaini, M. K., Dunlop, E. M. C., Emarah, M. H. M., Garland, J. A., Harper, A., Jones, B. R., Race, J. W., du Toit, M. S., Treharne, J. D. and Wright, D. J. M. (1966). Infection by TRIC agent and other members of the Bedsonia group. *Transactions of the Ophthalmological Society* **86**, 313–320.

Frei, W. (1925). Eine neue Hautreaktion bei Lymphogranuloma inguinale. *Klinische Wochenschrift* **4**, 2148–2149.

Friis, R. R. (1972). Interaction of L cells and *C. psittaci*: entry of the parasite and host responses to its development. *Journal of Bacteriology* **110**, 706–721.

Fritsch, H. O., Hofstatter, A. and Lindner, K. (1910). Experimentelle Studien zur Trachomfrage. *Graefe's Archiv fur Ophthalmologie* **76**, 547.

Frommell, G. T., Bruhn, F. W., and Schwartzman, J. D. (1977). Isolation of *C. trachomatis* from infant lung tissue. *New England Journal of Medicine* **296**, 1150–1152.

Frommell, G. T., Rothenberg, R., Wang, S-P. and McIntosh, K. (1979). Chlamydial infection of mothers and their infants. *Journal of Pediatrics* **95**, 28–32.

Furness, G., Graham, D. and Reeve, P. (1960). The titration of Trachoma and Inclusion Blennorrhea viruses in cell cultures. *Journal of General Microbiology* **23**, 613–619.

Gale, J. L., Chiang, W. T., Gordon, J. M. and Lai, J. S. (1970). Human genital infection with *Chlamydia* in Taiwan. *Journal of Formosan Medical Association* **69**, 610.

Gale, J. L., Di Giacomo, R. F., Kiviat, M. D., Wang, S. P. and Bowie, W. R. (1977). Experimental Non-human Primate Urethral Infection with *C. trachomatis* and *Ureaplasma*. In *Non-gonococcal Urethritis and Related Infections*, pp. 205–213. Edited by Hobson, D. and Holmes, K. K., American Society for Microbiology, Washington D.C.

Gale, J. L., Wang, S-P. and Grayston, J. T. (1971). Chronic trachoma in two Taiwan monkeys ten years after infection. In: Trachoma and Related Disorders, Edited by Nichols, R. L., *Excerpta Medica, Amsterdam*. pp. 489–493.

Gerloff, R. K. and Watson, R. O. (1967). The radioisotope precipitation test for Psittacosis group antibody. *American Journal of Ophthalmology*. Series 3, **63**, 1492–1498.

Ghadirian, F. D. and Robson, H. G. (1979). *C. trachomatis* genital infections. *British Journal of Venereal Diseases* **55**, 415–418.

Ghione, M., Brivio, R., Sanfilippo, A. and Schioppacassi, G. (1967). Research on factors influencing experimental chemotherapy tests in Trachoma. *American Journal of Ophthalmology* **63**, 547–551.

Goldmeier, D. and Darougar, S. (1977). Isolation of *C. trachomatis* from throat and rectum of homosexual men. *British Journal of Venereal Diseases* **53**, 184–185.

Gordon, F. B., Harper, I. A., Quan, A. L., Treharne, J. D., Dwyer, R. St.C. and Garland J. A. (1969). Detection of Chlamydia (Bedsonia) in certain infections of man. I Laboratory procedures, comparison of yolk-sac and cells. *Journal of Infectious Diseases* **120**, 451–462.

Gordon, F. B. and Quan, A. (1962). Drug susceptibilities of the Psittacosis and Trachoma agents. *Annals of the New York Academy of Sciences*, **981** 261–270.

Gordon, F. and Quan, A. L. (1965). Isolation of Trachoma Agent in Cell Culture. *Proceedings of the Society of Experimental Biology (New York)*, **118**, 354–359.

Gordon, F. B., Quan, A. L. (1971). Isolation of *Chlamydia trachomatis* from the human genital tract by cell culture: a summary. In: Trachoma and Related Disorders. Edited by Nichols, R. L. *Excerpta Medica, Amsterdam*, pp. 476–487.

Gordon, F.B., Quan, A. L., Steinman, T. I. and Philip, R. N. (1973). Chlamydial isolates from Reiter's Syndrome. *British Journal of Venereal Diseases*, **49**, 376–380.

Grayston, J. T. and Wang, S-P. (1975). New knowledge of chlamydiae and the diseases they cause. *Journal of Infectious Diseases* **132**, 87–105.

Greaves, A. B., Hilleman, M. R., Taggart, S. R., Bankhead, A. B. and Field, M. (1957). Chemotherapy in bubonic lymphogranuloma venereum: a clinical and serological evaluation. *Bulletin of the World Health Organisation* **16**, 277–289.

Greenblatt, R. B., Dienst, R. B. and Baldwin, K. R. (1959). Lymphogranuloma venereum and granuloma inguinale. *Medical Clinics of North America*, **43**, 1493–1506.

Halberstaedter, L. and von Prowazek, S. (1907). Über Zelleinschlüsse

Parasitärer Natur beim Trachom. *Arbeiten aus dem Kaiserlichen Gesundheitsamke* **26,** 44–47.

Hamark, B., Brorsson, J-E., Tönnes, E. and Forssman, L. (1976). Salpingitis and Chlamydia Subgroup A. *Acta Obstetrica et Gynecologica Scandinavia* **55,** 377–378.

Hammerschlag, M. R., Anderka, M., Semine, D. Z., McComb, D. and McCormack, W. M. (1979). Prospective study of maternal and infantile infections with *C. trachomatis. Pediatrics* **64,** 142–148.

Hammerschlag, M. R., Chandler, J. W., Alexander, E. R., English, M., Chiang, W-T., Koutsky, L., Eschenbach, D. A. and Smith, J. R. (1980). Erythromycin ointment for ocular prophylaxis of neonatal chlamydial infection. *Journal of the American Medical Association* **244,** 2291–3.

Handsfield, H. H., Alexander, E. R., Wang, S-P., Pedersen, A. H. B. and Holmes, K. K. (1976). Differences in the therapeutic response of chlamydia–positive and chlamydia–negative forms of non-gonococcal urethritis. *Journal of American Venereal Diseases Association* **2,** 5–9.

Hanna, L., Dawson, C. R., Briones, O., Thygeson, P. and Jawetz, E. (1968). Latency in human infections with TRIC agents. *Journal of Immunology* **101,** 43–50.

Hanna, L., Jawetz, E., Briones, O. C., Keshishyan, H., Hoshiwara, I., Bruce Ostler, H. and Dawson, C. R. (1973). Antibodies to TRIC agents in tears and serum of naturally infected humans. *Journal of Infectious Diseases* **27,** 95–98.

Hare, M. J., Taylor-Robinson, D., Oates, J. K., Evans, R.T., and Furr, P. M. (1980). *C. trachomatis* as a cause of follicular cervicitis. *Obstetrics and Gynaecology* (in press).

Harkness, A. H. (1950). Non-gonococcal urethritis. Livingstone, Edinburgh.

Harnisch, J. P., Berger, R. E., Alexander, E. R., Monda, G. and Holmes, K. K. (1977). Aetiology of acute epididymitis. *Lancet* **I,** 819–821.

Harper, I. A., Dwyer, R. St.C., Garland, J. A., Jones, B. R., Treharne, J. D., Dunlop, E. M. C., Freedman, A. and Race, J. W. (1967). Infection by Bedsoniae and the possibility of spurious isolation: 1. cross infection of eggs during culture. *American Journal of Ophthalmology* **63,** 1064–1073.

Harrison, H. R., Alexander, E. R., Chiang, W. T., Giddens, W. E., Boyce, J. T., Benjamin, D. and Gale, J. L. (1979). Experimental nasopharyngitis and pneumonia caused by *C. trachomatis* in infant baboons; histopathologic comparison with a case in a human infant. *Journal of Infectious Diseases* **139,** 141–146.

Harrison, H. R., English, M. G., Lee, C. K. and Alexander, E. R. (1978). *C. trachomatis* infant pneumonitis. *New England Journal of Medicine* **298,** 702–708.

Harrison, R. F., de Louvois, J. and Blades, M. (1975). Doxycycline treatment and human infertility. *Lancet* **I,** 605–607.

Hatch, T. P. (1975). Competition between *C. psittaci* and L cells for host isoleucine pools: a limiting factor in chlamydial multiplication. *Infection and Immunity* **12,** 211–219.

Heap, G. (1975). Acute epididymitis attributable to chlamydial infection — preliminary report. *Medical Journal of Australia* **1,** 718–719.

Heymann, B. (1910). Über die Fundorte der Powazetz'schen Körperchen. *Berliner Klinische Wochenschrift* **47**, 663–666.

Hilton, A. L., Richmond, S. J., Milne, J. D., Hindley, F. and Clarke, S. K. R. (1974). Chlamydia A in the female genital tract. *British Journal of Venereal Diseases* **50** 1–9

Hobson, D., Johnson, F. W. A., Rees, E. and Tait, I. A. (1974). Simplified method for diagnosis of genital and ocular infections with chlamydia. *Lancet* **II**, 555–556.

Hobson, D. and Rees, E. (1977). Chlamydial infection in neonates. *New England Journal of Medicine* **297**, 398.

Holmes, K. K., Handsfield, H. H., Wang, S-P., Wentworth, B. B., Turck, M., Anderson, J. B. and Alexander, E. R. (1975). Etiology of non-gonococcal urethritis. *New England Journal of Medicine* **292**, 1199–1206.

Holmes, K. K., Johnson, D. W. and Floyd, T. M. (1967). Studies of venereal disease III Double-blind comparison of tetracycline hydrochloride and placebo in treatment of non-gonococcal urethritis. *Journal of the American Medical Association* **202**, 474–476.

Holt, S., Pedersen, A. H. B., Wane, S. P., Kenny, G. E., Foy, H. M. and Grayston, J. T. (1967). Isolation of TRIC agents and mycoplasma from the genito-urinary tracts of patients of a venereal disease clinic. *American Journal of Ophthalmology* **63**, 1057–1064.

Howard, L. V., O'Leary, M. P. and Nichols, R. L. (1976). Animal model studies of genital chlamydial infections — immunity to reinfection with guinea-pig inclusion conjunctivitis agent in the urethra and eye of male guinea-pigs. *British Journal of Venereal Diseases* **52**, 261–265.

Hurst, E. W., Peters, J. M., Melvin, P. (1950). The therapy of experimental psittacosis and lymphogranuloma venereum (inguinale) 1. The comparative efficiency of penicillin, choramphenicol, aureomycin and terramycin. *British Journal of Pharmacology and Chemotherapy* **5**, 611–624.

Hutchinson, G. R., Taylor-Robinson, D. and Dourmashkin, R. R. (1979). Growth and effect of chlamydiae in human and bovine oviduct organ cultures. *British Journal of Venereal Diseases* **55**, 194–202.

Irons, J. V., Sullivan, T. D. and Rowen, J. (1951). Outbreaks of psittacosis from working with turkeys or chickens. *American Journal of Public Health* **41**; 931–937.

Jacobs, N. F., Arum, E. S. and Kraus, S. J. (1978). Experimental infection of the chimpanzee urethra and pharynx with *C. trachomatis. Sexually Transmitted Diseases* **5**, 132–136.

Jawetz, E. (1962). Seasonal insusceptibility of embryonated eggs to viruses of Trachoma and Inclusion conjunctivitis. *Annals of the New York Academy of Sciences* **98**, 31–37.

Jawetz, E. (1962). Discussion. *Annals of the New York Academy of Sciences* **98**, 278.

Jawetz, E. (1969). Chemotherapy of chlamydial infections. *Advances in Pharmacology and Chemotherapy* **12**, 253–282.

Jeffcoate, N. (1975). *Principles of gynaecology*, p. 315. Butterworths, London and Boston.

Johannisson, G., Edmar, B. and Lycke, E. (1977). *Chlamydia trachomatis* infections and venereal disease. *Acta dermato-venereologica* **57**, 455–458.

Johannisson, G., Sernryd, A. and Lycke, E. (1979). Susceptibility of *C. trachomatis* to antibiotics *in vitro* and *in vivo*. *Sexually Transmitted Diseases* **6,** 50–57.

Johnson, F. W. A., Chancerelle, L. Y. J. and Hobson, D. (1978). An improved method for demonstrating the growth of chlamydiae in tissue culture. *Medical Laboratory Sciences* **35,** 67–74.

Johnson, F. W. A. and Hobson, D. (1977). The effect of penicillin on genital strains of *C. trachomatis* in tissue culture. *Journal of Antimicrobial Chemotherapy* **3,** 49–56.

Johnston, P. B. (1962). Discussion. *Annals of the New York Academy of Sciences* **98,** 280.

Jones, B.R. (1964). Ocular syndromes of TRIC virus infection and their possible genital significance. *British Journal of Venereal Diseases* **40,** 3–18.

Jones, B. R. (1975). Prevention of blindness from trachoma. *Transactions of the Ophthalmological Society* **95,** 16–33.

Jones, B. R., Collier, L. H. and Smith, C. H. (1959). Isolation of virus from inclusion blennorrhoea. *Lancet* **I,** 902–905.

Jones, H., Rake, G. and Stearns, B. (1945). Studies on L.G.V. III *Journal of Infectious Diseases* **76,** 55–69.

Kazal, H. L., Sohn, N. and Corrasco, J. I. (1976). The gay bowel syndrome: clinico-pathologic correlation in 260 cases. *Annals of Clinical Laboratory Sciences* **6,** 184–192.

Keat, A. C., Maini, R. N., Nkwazi, G. C., Pegrum, G. D., Ridgway, G. L. and Scott, J. T. (1978). Role of *C. trachomatis* and HLA-B27 in sexually acquired reactive arthritis. *British Medical Journal* **1,** 605–607.

Keat, A. C., Thomas, B. J., Taylor-Robinson, D., Pegrum, G. D., Maini, R. N. and Scott, J. T. (1980). Evidence of *C. trachomatis* infection in sexually acquired reactive arthritis. *Annals of the Rheumatic Diseases* **39,** 431–437.

Kinsella, J. D., Norton, W. L. and Ziff, M. (1968). Complement-fixing antibodies to *Bedsonia* organisms in Reiter's syndrome and ankylosing spondylitis. *Annals of the Rheumatic Diseases* **27,** 241–244.

King, A. (1964). *Recent Advances in Venereology*, pp. 304–333. J. and A. Churchill Ltd, London.

Koch, R. (1883). Thatigkeit der Deutschen Cholerakommision in Aegypten und Ostundien. *Wiener Klinische Wochenschrift* **33,** 1550.

Kousa, M., Saikku, P., Richmond, S. and Lassus, A. (1978). Frequent associations of chlamydial infection with Reiter's syndrome. *Sexually Transmitted Diseases* **5,** 57–61.

Kramer, M. J. and Gordon, F. B. (1971). Ultrastructural analysis of the effects of penicillin and chlortetracycline on the development of a genital tract *Chlamydia*. *Infection and Immunity* **3,** 333–341.

Kroner, T. (1884). "Zur Aetiologie der Opthalmoblennorrhea Neonatorum". *Zentralblatt für Gynäkologie* **8,** 643.

Kuo, C-C and Chen, W. J. (1980). A mouse model of *C. trachomatis* pneumonitis. *Journal of Infectious Diseases* **141,** 198–202.

Kuo, C-C., Wang, S. and Grayston, J. T. (1978). Antimicrobial activity of several antibiotics and a sulfonamide against *C. trachomatis* organisms in cell culture. *Antimicrobial agents and Chemotherapy* **12,** 80–83.

Kuo, C-C., Wang, S-P., Wentworth, B. B. and Grayston, J. T. (1972).

Primary isolation of TRIC organisms in HeLa 229 cells treated with DEAE-Dextran. *Journal of Infectious Diseases* **125,** 665–668.

Law, W. A. (1943). Treatment of lymphogranuloma inguinale with anthiomaline. *Lancet* **I,** 300–304.

Lassus, A., Mustakiallio, K. K. and Wagner, O. (1970). Auto-immune serum factors and IgA elevation in lymphogranuloma venereum. *Annals of Clinical Research* **2,** 51–56.

Lee, C. K., Bowie, W. R. and Alexander, E. R. (1978). *In vitro* assays of the efficacy of antimicrobial agents in controlling *C. trachomatis* propagation. *Antimicrobial Agents and Chemotherapy* **13,** 441–445.

Levin, I., Romano, S., Steinberg, M. and Welsh, R. A. (1964). Lymphogranuloma venereum: rectal stricture and carcinoma. *Diseases of the Colon and Rectum* **7,** 129–134.

Lewis, V. J., Thacker, W. L. and Mitchell, S. (1977). ELISA for chlamydial antibodies. *Journal of Clinical Microbiology* **6,** 507–510.

Lindner, K. (1909). Uebertragungsversuche von gonokokkenfreier Blennorrhea neonatorum auf Affen. *Wiener Klinische Wochenschrift* **22,** 1554–1659.

Lycke, E., Lowhagen, G-B., Hallhagen, G., Johannisson, G. and Ramstedt, K. (1980). The risk of transmissions of genital *C. trachomatis* infection is less than that of genital *Neisseria gonorrhoeae* infection. *Sexually Transmitted Diseases* **7,** 6–10.

McComb, D. E., Nichols, R. L., Semine, D. Z., Everard, J. R., Alpert, S., Crockett, V. A., Rosner, B., Zinner, S. H. and McCormack, W. M. (1979). *C. trachomatis* in women: antibody in cervical secretions as a possible indication of genital infection. *Journal of Infectious Diseases* **139,** 628–633.

McCormack, W. M., Alpert, S., McComb, D. E., Nichols, R. L., Semine, Z. and Zinner, S. H. (1979). Fifteen-month follow-up study of women infected with *C. trachomatis*. *New England Journal of Medicine* **300,** 123–125.

Majčuk, J. (1976). Trachoma control in the eastern mediterranean region. *World Health Organisation Chronical* **30,** 97–100.

Manire, G. P. (1977). Biological characteristics of Chlamydia. In *Non-gonococcal urethritis and related infections*, p. 167–175. Edited by Hobson, D. and Holmes, K. K. American Society for Microbiology, Washington DC.

Manire, G. P. and Galasso, G. J. (1959). Persistent infection of HeLa cells with meningo-pneumonitis virus. *Journal of Immunology* **83,** 529–533.

Mårdh, P-A (1975). Proceedings of the symposium. In *Genital infections and their complications*, p. 209. Edited by Danielsson, D., Juhlin, L. and Mårdh, P-A. Almqvist and Wiksell International. Stockholm, Sweden.

Mårdh, P-A., Helin, I., Bobeck, S., Lavrin, J. and Nilsson, T. (1980). Colonisation of pregnant and puerperal women and neonates with *C. trachomatis*. *British Journal of Venereal Diseases* **56,** 96–100.

Mårdh, P-A., Ripa, K. T., Colleen, S., Treharne, J. D. and Darougar, S. (1978). Role of *C. trachomatis* in non-acute prostatitis. *British Journal of Venereal Diseases* **54,** 330–334.

Mårdh, P-A., Ripa, K. T., Svensson, L. and Weström, L. (1977). *C. trachomatis* infection in patients with acute salpingitis. *New England Journal of Medicine* **296,** 1377–1379.

Martin, D. H., Alexander, E. R., Eschenbach, D. A., Kuo, C. C., Chaing, W. T., Maclurg, B. J., Adam, J., Koutsky, L. and Holmes, K. K. (1979). Prospective study of *Chlamydia* infections in pregnancy. *Journal of Clinical*

Research **27,** 479.

Menke, H. E., Schuller, J. L. and Stolz, E. (1979). Treatment of lymphogranuloma venereum with rifampicin. *British Journal of Venereal Diseases* **55,** 379.

Meyer, K. F. (1953). Psittacosis group. *Annals of the New York Academy of Sciences* **56,** 515–556.

Meyer, K. F. and Eddie, B. (1951). Human carrier of the Psittacosis virus. *Journal of Infectious Diseases* **88,** 109–125.

Meyer, K. F. and Eddie, B. (1964). Psittacosis-lymphogranuloma venereum group (Bedsonia infection). In *Diagnostic procedures for Viral and Rickettsial Diseases*, 3rd Edition, Chapter 22, p. 603. Edited by Lennette, E. and Schmidt, N. American Public Health Association, Inc., New York.

Miles, R. P. M. (1957). Rectal lymphogranuloma venereum. *British Journal of Surgery* **45,** 180–188.

Miles, R. P. M. (1959). Rectal lymphogranuloma venereum. *Postgraduate Medical Journal* **35,** 92–96.

Møller, B. R., Mårdh, P-A. (1980). Experimental salpingitis in grivet monkeys by *C. trachomatis*. *Acta pathologica et microbiologica Scandinavia*, Section B **88,** 107–114.

Møller, B. R., Weström, L., Ahrons, S., Ripa, K. T., Svensson, L., von Mecklenburg, C., Henrickson, H. and Mårdh, P-A. (1979). *C. trachomatis* infections of the fallopian tubes. Histological findings in two patients. *British Journal of Venereal Diseases* **55,** 422–428.

Moulder, J. W. (1964). *The psittacosis group as bacteria. Ciba lectures in Microbiology and Biochemistry*, Wiley, New York.

Moulder, J. W. (1966). The relation of the psittacosis group (chlamydia) to bacteria and viruses. *Annual Review of Microbiology* **20,** 107–130.

Mount, D. T., Bigazzi, P. E. and Barron, A. L. (1973). Experimental genital infection of male guinea-pigs with the agent of guinea-pig inclusion conjunctivitis and transmission to females. *Infection and Immunity* **8,** 925–930.

Müller-Schoop, J. W., Wang, S-P., Munzinger, J., Schläpfer, H. V., Knoblaugh, M. and Ammann, R. W. (1978). *C. trachomatis* as a possible cause of peritonitis and perihepatitis in young women. *British Medical Journal* **1,** 1022–1024.

Munday, P. E., Johnson, A. P., Thomas, B. J. and Taylor-Robinson, D. (1980). A comparison of the sensitivity of immunofluorescence and Giemsa for staining cycloheximide-treated McCoy cells. *Journal of Clinical Pathology* **33,** 177–179.

Munro, J., Mayberry, J. F., Matthews, N. and Rhodes, J. (1979). Chlamydia and Chrohn's disease. *Lancet* **II,** 45–46.

Murray, E. S. (1977). Review of clinical, epidemiological and immunological studies of guinea pig inclusion conjunctivitis infection in guinea-pigs. In *Non-gonococcal urethritis and related infections*, p. 199. Edited by Hobson, D. and Holmes, K. K. American Society for Microbiology, Washington DC.

Nabli, B. and Tarizzo, M. L. (1967). The effect of antiseptics and other substances on TRIC agents. *American Journal of Ophthalmology* **63,** 515–524.

Naib, Z. M. (1970). Cytology of TRIC agent infection of the eye of newborn infants and their mothers' genital tracts. *Acta Cytologica* (Baltimore) **14,** 390–395.

Nayyar, K. C., O'Neill, J. J., Hambling, M. H. and Waugh, M. A. (1976). Isolation of *C. trachomatis* from women attending a clinic for sexually transmitted diseases. *British Journal of Venereal Diseases* **52,** 396–398.

Officer, J. E. and Brown, A. (1961). Serial changes in virus and cells in cultures chronically infected with psittacosis virus. *Virology* **14,** 88–89.

Oriel, J. D., Johnson, A. L., Barlow, D., Thomas, B. J., Nayyar, K. and Reeve, P. (1978). Infection of the uterine cervix with *C. trachomatis*. *Journal of Infectious Diseases* **137,** 443–451.

Oriel, J. D., Powis, P. A., Reeve, P., Miller, A. and Nicol, C. S. (1974). Chlamydial infections of the cervix. *British Journal of Venereal Diseases* **50,** 11–16.

Oriel, J. D., Reeve, P. and Nicol, C. S. (1975a). Minocycline in the treatment of non-gonococcal urethritis: its effect on *C. trachomatis*. *Journal of American Venereal Disease Association* **2,** 17–22.

Oriel, J. D., Reeve, P., Thomas, B. J. and Nicol, C. S. (1975b). Infection with *Chlamydia* Group A in men with urethritis due to *Neisseria gonorrhoeae*. *Journal of Infectious Diseases* **131,** 376–382.

Oriel, J. D., Reeve, P., Powis, P. A., Miller, A. and Nicol, C. S. (1972). Chlamydial infection: isolation of *Chlamydia* from patients with non-specific genital infection. *British Journal of Venereal Diseases* **48,** 429–436.

Oriel, J. D., Reeve, P., Wright, J. T. and Owen, J. (1976). Chlamydial infection of the male urethra. *British Journal of Venereal Diseases* **52,** 46–51.

Oriel, J. D. and Ridgway, G. L. (1980). Comparison of erythromycin and oxytetracycline in the treatment of cervical infection by *C. trachomatis*. *Journal of Infection* **2,** 259–262.

Oriel, J. D., Ridgway, G. L., Reeve, P., Beckinham, D. C. and Owen, J. (1976). The lack of effect of ampicillin plus probenecid given for genital infections with *Neisseria gonorrhoeae* on associated infections with *C. trachomatis*. *Journal of Infectious Diseases* **133,** 568–571.

Oriel, J. D., Ridgway, G. L. and Tchamouroff, S. (1977a). Comparison of erythromycin stearate and oxytetracycline in the treatment of non-gonococcal urethritis: their efficacy against *C. trachomatis*. *Scottish Medical Journal* **22,** 375–379.

Oriel, J. D., Ridgway, G. L., Tchamouroff, S. and Owen, J. (1977b). Spectinomycin hydrochloride in the treatment of gonorrhoea: its effect on associated *C. trachomatis* infections. *British Journal of Venereal Diseases* **53,** 226–229.

Paavonen, J. (1979). *C. trachomatis* induced urethritis in female partners of men with non-gonococcal urethritis. *Sexually Transmitted Diseases* **6,** 69–71.

Paavonen, J., Kousa, M., Saikku, P. A., Vartianen, E., Kanerva, L. and Lassus, A. (1980). Treatment of non-gonococcal urethritis with trimethoprim sulphadiazine and with placebo. *British Journal of Venereal Diseases* **56,** 101–104.

Paavonen, J., Kousa, M., Saikku, P., Vesterinen, E., Jansson, E. and Lassus, A. (1978a). Examination of men with non-gonococcal urethritis and their sexual partners for *C. trachomatis* and *Ureaplasma urealyticum*. *Sexually Transmitted Diseases* **5,** 93–96.

Paavonen, J., Saikku, P., Vesterinen, E., Meyer, B., Vartianen, E. and

Saksela, E. (1978b). Genital chlamydial infections in patients attending a gynaecological outpatient clinic. *British Journal of Venereal Diseases* **54**, 257–261.

Paavonen, J., Vesterinen, E., Meyer, B., Saikku, P., Suni, J., Purola, E. and Saksela, E. (1979a) Genital *C. trachomatis* infections in patients with cervical atypic. *Obstetrics and Gynecology* **54**, 289–291.

Paavonen, J. A., Saikku, P., Vesterinen, E. and Lehtovirta, P. (1979b). Infertility and cervical *C. trachomatis* infections. *Acta obstetrica et gynecologica Scandinavia* **58**, 301–303.

Paavonen, J.A., Saikku, P., Vesterinen, E. and Aho, K. (1979c). *C. trachomatis* in acute salpingitis. *British Journal of Venereal Diseases* **55**, 203–206.

Page, L. A. (1966). Revision of the family *Chlamydiaceae* (Rake) *International Journal of Systematic Bacteriology* **16**, 223–252.

Page, L. A. (1968). Proposal for the recognition of two species in the genus Chlamydia. *International Journal of Systematic Bacteriology* **18**, 51–66.

Perroud, H. M. and Miedzybrodzka, K. (1978). Chlamydial infection of the urethra in men. *British Journal of Venereal Diseases* **54**, 45–49.

Philip, R. N., Hill, D. A., Greaves, A. B., Gordon, F. B., Quan, A. L., Gerloff, R. K. and Thomas, L. A. (1971). Study of Chlamydiae in patients with LGV and urethritis attending a V.D. clinic. *British Journal of Venereal Diseases* **47**, 114–121.

Prentice, M. J., Taylor-Robinson, D. and Csonka, G. W. (1976). Non-specific urethritis. A placebo-controlled trial of minocycline in conjunction with laboratory investigations. *British Journal of Venereal Diseases* **52**, 269–275.

Pund, E. R. and Lacy, G. R. (1951). Lymphogranuloma venereum (inguinale), a precipitating cause of carcinoma. Statistical analysis of one hundred and thirty five cases of carcinoma of penis, vulva and anorectum. *American Surgeon* **17**, 711–718.

Rainey, R. (1954). The association of lymphogranuloma inguinale and cancer. *Surgery* **35**, 221–235.

Rees, E., Tait, I. A., Hobson, D. and Johnson, R. W. A. (1977a). Chlamydia in relation to cervical and pelvic inflammatory disease. In *Non-gonococcal urethritis and related infections*, p. 67–76. Edited by Hobson, D. and Holmes, K. K. American Society for Microbiology, Washington DC.

Rees, E., Tait, I. A., Hobson, D. and Johnson, F. W. A. (1977b). Perinatal chlamydial infection. In *Non-gonococcal urethritis and related infections*, p. 140–147. Edited by Hobson, D. and Holmes, K. K. American Society for Microbiology, Washington DC.

Rees, E., Tait, I. A., Hobson, D., Byng, R. E. and Johnson, F. W. A. (1977c). Neonatal conjunctivitis caused by *N. gonorrhoeae* and *C. trachomatis*. *British Journal of Venereal Diseases* **53**, 173–179.

Reeve, P. (1976). The inactivation of *C. trachomatis* by povidone iodine. *Journal of Antimicrobial Chemotherapy* **2**, 77–81.

Reeve, P., Gerloff, R. K., Casper, E., Philip, R. N., Oriel, J. D. and Powis, P. A. (1974). Serological studies on the role of *Chlamydia* in the aetiology of non-specific urethritis. *British Journal of Venereal Diseases* **50**, 136–139.

Reeve, P., Owen, J. and Oriel, J. D. (1975). Laboratory procedures for the isolation of *C. trachomatis* from the human genital tract. *Journal of Clinical Pathology* **28**, 910–914.

Reeve, P., Taverne, J. and Bushby, S. R. M. (1968). Inhibition by pyrimidine analogues of the synthesis of folic acid by trachoma agents. *Journal of Hygiene Cambridge* **66**, 295–308.

Richmond, S. J. (1976). Growth of *C. trachomatis* in cell culture. *Lancet* **I**, 865.

Richmond, S. J. and Caul, E. O., (1975). Fluorescent antibody studies in chlamydial infection. *Journal of Clinical Microbiology* **1**, 345–352.

Richmond, S. J. and Caul, E. O. (1977). Single-antigen indirect immuno-fluorescence test for screening venereal disease clinic populations for chlamydial antibodies. In *Non-gonococcal urethritis and related infections*, p. 259–265. Edited by Hobson, D. and Holmes, K. K. American Society for Microbiology, Washington DC.

Richmond, S. J., Hilton, A. L. and Clarke, S. K. R. (1972). Chlamydial infection. Role of *Chlamydia* Sub-group A in non-gonococcal and post-gonococcal urethritis. *British Journal of Venereal Diseases* **48**, 437–444.

Richmond, S. J., Milne, J. D., Hilton, A. L. and Caul, E. O. (1980). Antibodies to *C. trachomatis* in cervicovaginal secretions: relation to serum antibodies and current chlamydial infection. *Sexually Transmitted Diseases* **7**, 11–15.

Richmond, S. J. and Oriel, J. D. (1978). Recognition and management of genital chlamydial infection. *British Medical Journal* **2**, 480–483.

Richmond, S. J., Paul, I. D. and Taylor, P. K. (1980). Value and feasibility of screening women attending STD clinics for cervical chlamydial infections. *British Journal of Venereal Diseases*, **56**, 92–95.

Richmond, S. J. and Sparling, P. F. (1976). Genital chlamydial infections. *American Journal of Epidemiology* **103**, 428–435.

Ridgway, G. L. (1982). Chlamydia trachomatis. In *Laboratory methods in antimicrobial chemotherapy* 2nd edition. Edited by Reeves, D. S., Phillips, I., Williams, J. D. and Wise, R. Churchill Livingstone (In press).

Ridgway, G. L., Boulding, S., Lam Po Tang, V. (1980). The activity of rifamycins against *C. trachomatis in vitro*. In *Current Chemotherapy and infectious diseases*, p. 1275. (Proceedings of the 11th International Congress of Chemotherapy and the 19th Interscience Conference on antimicrobial agents and chemotherapy); Edited by Nelson, J. D. and Grassi, C. American Society for Microbiology.

Ridgway, G. L. and Oriel, J. D. (1977a). Interrelationship of *C. trachomatis* and other pathogens in the female genital tract. *Journal of Clinical Pathology* **30**, 933–936.

Ridgway, G. L. and Oriel, J. D. (1977b). Treatment of neonatal inclusion blennorrhea. *New England Journal of Medicine* **297**, 512.

Ridgway, G. L., Owen, J. M. and Oriel, J D. (1976). A method for testing the antibiotic susceptibility of *C. trachomatis in a cell culture system*. *Journal of Antimicrobial Chemotherapy* **2**, 77–81.

Ripa, K. T. and Mårdh, P. A. (1977). Cultivation of *C. trachomatis* in cyclo-heximide-treated McCoy cells. *Journal of Clinical Microbiology* **6**, 328–331.

Ripa, T. K., Møller, B. R., Mårdh, P-A., Freundt, E. A. and Melsen, F. (1979). Experimental acute salpingitis in grivet monkeys provoked by *C. trachomatis*. *Acta pathologica et microbiologica Scandinavia*, Section B **87**, 65–70.

Ripa, K. T., Svensson, L., Mårdh, P-A. and Weström, L. (1978). *C. trachomatis* cervicitis in gynaecologic outpatients. *Obstetrics and Gynecology* **52**, 698–701.

Rodin, P. (1971). Asymptomatic non-specific urethritis. *British Journal of Venereal Diseases* **47,** 452–453.

Rota, T. and Nichols, R. (1971). Infection of cell culture by Trachoma agent: Enhancement by D.E.A.E. Dextran. *Journal of Infectious Diseases* **124,** 419–420.

Saad, E. A., de Gouveia, O. F., Dias, L. B. and da Silva, R. (1961). Alterazione delle proteini seriche e dell'istologia epatica della fase tardiva del linfo-granuloma venereo. *Archiv Italiano della Scienzia e della Medizini Tropicale.*

Sagy, M., Barzilay, Z. Yahav, J., Ginsberg, R. and Sompolinsky, D. (1980). Severe neonatal chlamydial pneumonitis. *American Journal of Diseases in Children* **134,** 89–90.

Saikku, P. and Paavonen, J. (1978). Single antigen immunofluorescence test for chlamydial antibodies. *Journal of Clinical Microbiology* **8,** 119–122.

Salari, S. H. and Ward, M. E. (1979). Early detection of *C. trachomatis* using fluorescent DNA binding dyes. *Journal of Clinical Pathology* **32,** 1155–1162.

Schachter, J. (1967). Isolation of *Bedsoniae* from human arthritis and abortion tissues. *American Journal of Ophthalmology* **63,** 1082–1086.

Schachter, J. (1971). Complement fixing antibodies to Bedsonia in Reiter's syndrome, TRIC agent infection and control groups. *American Journal of Ophthalmology* **71,** 857–860.

Schachter, J. (1976). In *Infection and immunology in the rheumatic diseases,* p. 147–150. Edited by Dumonde, D. C., Blackwell Scientific Publications, Oxford.

Schachter, J. (1978). Chlamydial infections. *New England Journal of Medicine,* **298,** 428–435; 490–495; 540–549.

Schachter, J. and Atwood, G. (1975). Chlamydial pharyngitis? *Journal of Americal Venereal Disease Association* **2,** 12.

Schachter, J., Barnes, M. G., Jones, J. P., Engleman, E. P. and Meyer, K. F. (1966). Isolation of Bedsoniae from the joints of patients with Reiter's syndrome. *Proceedings of the Society of Experimental Biology and Medicine* **122,** 283–285.

Schachter, J., Cles, L., Ray, R. and Hines, P. A. (1979a). Failure of serology in diagnosing chlamydial infections of the female genital tract. *Journal of Clinical Microbiology* **10,** 647–649.

Schachter, J. Grossman, M., Holt, J., Sweet, R. and Spector, S. (1979b). Infection with *C. trachomatis*: involvement of multiple anatomic sites in neonates. *Journal of Infectious Diseases* **139,** 232–234.

Schachter, J., Grossman, M., Holt, J., Sweet, R., Goodner, E. and Mills, J. (1979c). Prospective study of chlamydial infection in neonates. *Lancet* **II,** 377–379.

Schachter, J. and Dawson, C. R. (1977). Comparative efficiency of various diagnostic methods for chlamydial infection. *Non-gonococcal urethritis and related infections,* p. 337–341. Edited by Hobson, D. and Holmes, K. K. American Society for Microbiology, Washington DC.

Schachter, J., and Dawson, C. R. (1978). *Human chlamydial infections,* Chapter 11, p. 122. PSG Publishing Company Inc., Littleton, Massachusetts.

Schachter, J., Dawson, C. R., Balas, J. and Jones, P. (1970). Evaluation of laboratory methods for detecting acute TRIC agent infection. *American Journal of Ophthalmology* **70,** 375–380.

Schachter, J., Hanna, L., Hill, E. C., Massad, S., Sheppard, C. W., Conte, J. E., Cohen, S. N. and Meyer, K. F. (1975a). Are chlamydial infections the most prevalent venereal disease? *Journal of the American Medical Association* **231,** 1252–1255.

Schachter, J., Hill, E. C., King, E. B., Coleman, V. R., Jones, P. and Meyer, K. F. (1975b). Chlamydial infection in women with cervical dysplasia. *American Journal of Obstetrics and Gynaecology* **123,** 753–757.

Schachter, J., Lum, L., Gooding, C. A. and Ostler, B. (1975c). Pneumonitis following inclusion blennorrhea. *Journal of Pediatrics* **87,** 779–780.

Schachter, J., Rose, L., Dawson, C. R. and Barnes, M. (1967). Comparison of procedures for laboratory diagnosis of oculogenital infections with inclusion conjunctivitis agents. *American Journal of Epidemiology* **85,** 3, 453–458.

Schachter, J., Smith, A. E., Dawson, C. R., Anderson, W. R., Deller, J. J., Hoke, A. W., Smartt, W. H. and Meyer, K. F. (1969). Comparison of Frei test. Complement fixation test and isolation of the agent. *Journal of Infectious Diseases* **120,** 372–375.

Schuller, J. L., Piket-van Ulsen, J., Veeken, N. D., Michel, M. F. and Stolz, E. (1979). Antibodies against chlamydiae of lymphogranuloma venereum type in Crohn's disease. *Lancet* **I,** 19–20.

Sharp, J. T., Lidsky, M. D. and Riley, W. A. (1968). Clinical studies on gonococcal arthritis and Reiter's syndrome and measurement of gonococcal and Bedsonia antibodies. *Arthritis and Rheumatism* **11,** 569–578.

Sheldon, W. H. and Heyman, A. (1947). Lymphogranuloma venereum. A histologic study of the primary lesion, bubonulus and lymph nodes in cases proved by isolation of the virus. *American Journal of Pathology* **23,** 653–665.

Shiao, L., Wang, S. P. and Grayston, J. (1967). Sensitivity and Resistance of TRIC agents to Penicillin, Tetracycline and Sulpha drugs. *American Journal of Ophthalmology* **63,** 532–542.

Siboulet, A. and Galistin, P. (1962). Arguments in favour of a virus aetiology of non-gonococcal urethritis illustrated by three cases of Reiter's disease. *British Journal of Venereal Diseases* **38,** 209–211.

Simmons, P. D., Forsey, T., Thin, R. N., Treharne, J. D., Darougar, S., Langlet, F. and Pandhi, R. K. (1979). Antichlamydial antibodies in pelvic inflammatory disease. *British Journal of Venereal Diseases* **55,** 419–424.

Sompolinsky, D. and Richmond, S. J. (1974). Growth of *C. trachomatis* in McCoy cells treated with cytochalasin B. *Applied Microbiology* **28,** 912–914.

Sowa, J. and Race, M. W. (1971). Sensitivity of trachoma agent to streptomycin and other related antibiotics. *Journal of Hygiene* **69,** 709–716.

Stamm, W. E., Wagner, K. F., Amsel, R., Alexander, E. R., Turck, M., Counti, G. W. and Holmes, K. K. (1980). Etiology of the acute urethral syndrome in women. *New England Journal of Medicine* **303,** 409–415.

Storz, J. (1971). *Chlamydia and Chlamydia-induced diseases*. Charles C Thomas, Springfield, Illinois.

Swanson, J., Eschenbach, D. A., Alexander, E. R. and Holmes, K. K. (1975). Light-electronmicroscopic study of *C. trachomatis* infection of the uterine cervix. *Journal of Infectious Diseases* **131,** 678–687.

Swarbrick, E. T., Kingham, J. G. C., Price, H. C., Blackshaw, A. J., Griffiths, P. D., Darougar, S. and Buckell, N. A. (1979). Chlamydia, cytomegalovirus and Yersinia in inflammatory bowel disease. *Lancet* **II**, 11–12.

Swartz, S. L., Kraus, S. J., Herrmann, K. L., Stargel, M. D., Brown, W. J. and Allen, S. D. (1978). Diagnosis and etiology of non-gonococcal urethritis. *Journal of Infectious Diseases* **138**, 445–454.

Sweet, R. L., Mills, J., Hadley, K. W., Blumenstock, E., Schachter, J. Robbie, M. O. and Draper, D. L. (1980). Use of laparoscopy to determine the microbiologic etiology of acute salpingitis. *American Journal of Obstetrics and Gynecology* **134**, 68–74.

Tack, K. J., Peterson, P. K., Rasp, F. L., O'Leary, M., Hanto, D., Simmons, R. L. and Sabath, L. D. (1980). Isolation of *C. trachomatis* from the lower respiratory tract of adults. *Lancet* **I**, 116–117.

Tait, I. A., Rees, E., Hobson, D., Byng, R. E. and Tweedie, M. C. K. (1980). Chlamydial infection of the cervix in contacts of men with non-gonococcal urethritis. *British Journal of Venereal Diseases* **56**, 37–45.

Tait, I. A., Rees, E. and Jameson, R. M. (1978). Urethral syndrome associated with chlamydial infection of the urethra and cervix. *British Journal of Urology* **50**, 425.

T'ang, F. F., Chang, H. L., Huang, Y. T. and Wang, K. C. (1957). Studies on the aetiology of trachoma with special reference to isolation of the virus in chick embryo. *Chinese Medical Journal* **75**, 429–447.

Tarizzo, M. L. and Nabli, B. (1967). The effect of antibiotics on the growth of TRIC agents in embryonated eggs. *American Journal of Ophthalmology* **63**, 524–531.

Taylor-Robinson, D. and Munday, P. E. (1980). Chlamydia culture service. *British Journal of Venereal Diseases* **56**, 183.

Taylor-Robinson, D., O'Morain, C. A., Thomas, B. J. and Levi, A. J. (1979). Low frequency of chlamydial antibodies in patients with Crohn's disease and ulcerative colitis. *Lancet* **I**, 1162–1163.

Taylor-Robinson, D. and Thomas, B. J. (1980). The role of *C. trachomatis* in genital-tract and associated diseases. *Journal of Clinical Pathology* **33**, 205–233.

Terho, P. (1978a). *C. trachomatis* in non-specific urethritis. *British Journal of Venereal Diseases* **54**, 251–256.

Terho, P. (1978b). *Chlamydia trachomatis* in gonococcal and post-gonococcal urethritis. *British Journal of Venereal Diseases* **54**, 326–329.

Thomas, B. J., Reeve, P. and Oriel, J. D. (1976). Simplified serological test for antibodies to *C. trachomatis*. *Journal of Clinical Microbiology* **4**, 6–10.

Thompson, S. E. and Hager, W. D. (1977). Acute pelvic inflammatory disease. *Sexually Transmitted Diseases* **4**, 105–113.

Thygeson, P. and Mengert, W. F. (1936). The virus of inclusion conjunctivitis. Further observations. *Archives of Ophthalmology* **15**, 377–410.

Thygeson, P. and Stone, W. (1942). Epidemiology of inclusion conjunctivitis. *Archives of Ophthalmology* **27**, 91–122.

Tipple, M. A., Beem, M. O. and Saxon, E. M. (1979). Clinical characteristics of the afebrile pneumonia associated with *C. trachomatis* infection in infants under 6 months old. *Pediatrics* **63**, 192–197.

Treharne, J. D., Darougar, S. and Jones, B. R. (1977). Modification of the MIF test to provide a routine serodiagnostic test for chlamydial infection. *Journal of Clinical Pathology* **30**, 510–517.

Treharne, J. D., Darougar, S., Simmons, P. D. and Thin, R. N. (1978). Rapid diagnosis of chlamydial infection of the cervix. *British Journal of Venereal Diseases* **54**, 403–408.

Treharne, J. D., Day, J., Yeo, C. K., Jones, B. R. and Squires, S. (1977). Susceptibility of Chlamydiae to Chemotherapeutic Agents. In *Non-gonococcal urethritis and related infections*, pp. 214–222. Edited by Hobson, D. and Holmes, K. K. American Society for Microbiology, Washington DC.

Treharne, J. D., Ripa, K. T., Mårdh, P-A., Svensson, L., Weström, L. and Darougar, S. (1979). Antibodies to *C. trachomatis* in acute salpingitis. *British Journal of Venereal Diseases* **55**, 26–29.

Van der Bel-Khan, J. M., Watanakunakorn, C., Menefee, M. G., Long, H. D. and Dicter, R. (1978). *C. trachomatis* endocarditis. *American Heart Journal* **95**, 627–636.

Vaughan-Jackson, J. D., Dunlop, E. M. C., Darougar, S., Dwyer, R. St.C. and Jones, B. R. (1972). Chlamydial infection. Results of tests for *Chlamydia* in patients suffering from acute Reiter's disease compared with results of tests of the genital tract and rectum in patients with ocular infections due to TRIC agent. *British Journal of Venereal Diseases* **48**, 445–451.

Vaughan-Jackson, J. D., Dunlop, E. M. C., Darougar, S., Treharne, J. D. and Taylor-Robinson, D. (1977). Urethritis due to *C. trachomatis*. *British Journal of Venereal Diseases* **53**, 180–183.

von Wahl, A. (1911). *Deutsche Medizinische Wochenschrift* **37**, 118.

Wachtel, E. G. (1969). *Exfoliative cytology in gynaecological practice, 2nd edition* p. 148. Butterworth, London.

Wang, S. P. (1971). A micro-immunofluorescence method. Study of antibody response to TRIC organisms in mice. In: *Trachoma and related disorders caused by chlamydial agents*, p. 273–288. Edited by Nichol, R. L. Excerpta Medica, Amsterdam.

Wang, S-P and Grayston, J. T. (1970). Immunologic relationship between genital TRIC, lymphogranuloma venereum and related organisms in a new microtiter indirect immunofluorescence test. *American Journal of Ophthalmology* **70**, 367–374.

Wang, S-P. and Grayston, J. T. (1971). Local systemic antibody response to trachoma infection in monkeys. In: *Trachoma and Related disorders caused by chlamydial agents*. Edited by Nichols, R. L. Excerpta Medica, Amsterdam. p. 217–232.

Wang, S-P, and Grayston, J. T. (1974). Human serology in *C. trachomatis* infection with microimmunofluorescence. *Journal of Infectious Diseases* **130**, 388–397.

Wang, S-P., Grayston, J. T., Alexander, E. R. and Holmes, K. K. (1975). Simplified microimmunofluorescence test with Trachoma—LGV (*C. trachomatis*) antigen for use as a screening test for antibody. *Journal of Clinical Microbiology* **1**, 250–255.

Wang, S-P., Grayston, J. T., Kuo, C-C., Alexander, E. R. and Holmes, K. K. (1977). Serodiagnosis of *C. trachomatis* infection with the micro-immunofluorescence test. In *Non-gonococcal urethritis and related infections*, p. 237. Edited by Hobson, D. and Holmes, K. K. American Society for Microbiology, Washington DC.

Ward, M. E., Watt, P. J. and Robertson, J. N. (1974). The human fallopian tube: a laboratory model for gonococcal infection. *Journal of Infectious Diseases* **129,** 650–659.

Watson, P. G. and Gairdner, D. (1968). TRIC agent as a cause of neonatal eye sepsis. *British Medical Journal,* **2,** 527–528.

Waugh, M. A. and Nayyar, K. C. (1977). Triple tetracycline (Deteclo) in the treatment of chlamydial infection of the female genital tract. *British Journal of Venereal Diseases* **53,** 96–97.

Weiss, E., Myers, W. F., Dressler, H. R. and Chun-hoon, H. (1964). Glucose metabolism by agents of the Psittacosis-trachoma group. *Virology* **22,** 551–62.

Wentworth, B. and Alexander, E. R. (1974). The use of IUDR-treated cells for the isolation of *C. trachomatis. Applied Microbiology* **27,** 912–916.

Wentworth, B. B., Bonin, P., Holmes, K. K., Gutman, L., Wiesner, P. and Alexander, E. R. (1973). Isolation of viruses, bacteria and other organisms from venereal disease clinics and patients: methodology and problems associated with multiple isolations. *Health Laboratory Sciences* **10,** 75–81.

Werner, G. H. (1961). Recherches Expérimentales sur la Chimotherapie Du Trachome. *Annales de L'Institut Pasteur* **100,** 93–108.

Willcox, J. R., Fisk, P. G., Barrow, J. and Barlow, D. (1979). The need for a chlamydial culture service. *British Journal of Venereal Diseases* **55,** 281–283.

Wølner-Hanssen, P. Weström, L. and Mårdh, P-A. (1980). Perihepatitis and chlamydial salpingitis. *Lancet* **I,** 901–903.

Wong, J. L., Hines, P. A., Brasher, M. D., Rogers, G. T., Smith, R. F. and Schachter, J. (1977). The etiology of non-gonococcal urethritis in men attending a venereal disease clinic. *Sexually Transmitted Diseases* **4,** 4–8.

Woolfitt, J. M. G. and Watt, L., (1977). Chlamydial infection of the urogenital tract in promiscuous and non-promiscuous women. *British Journal of Venereal Diseases* **53,** 93–95.

Yong, E. C., Chinn, J. S., Caldwell, H. D. and Kuo, C-C. (1979). Reticulate bodies as single antigen in *C. trachomatis* with micro-immunofluorescence. *Journal of Clinical Microbiology* **10,** 351–356.

Index

Index